FINDING GOD

IN THE MIDDLE OF THE

FOOD WARS

Getting Healthy at the Cellular Level & Becoming What God Created "You" to Be!

Dr. Francis Myles • Coach Scott Oatsvall

FINDING GOD IN THE MIDDLE OF FOOD WARS

Published by Dr. Francis Myles and Scott Oatsvall

Library of Congress Cataloging-in-Publication Data:

An application to register this book for cataloging has been submitted to the Library of Congress.

International Standard Book Number: E-book ISBN:

Printed in the United States of America

MY DEEPEST APPRECIATION TO...

First and foremost, I want to thank God for His grace and His showers of blessings throughout my life's work and research on this project.

A special "Thank You" to my wife Gwen and our six children for all of their love and unwavering support. I would also like to express my deep and sincere gratitude to Dr. Jae Hitson, my staff, and the team at LT360 with a special "thank you" to Coach Ken Brooks, a guest writer on many of the chapters.

Finally, a thank you to Dr. Francis Myles for his friendship, wisdom, and partnership on this project. I am extending my heartfelt thanks to his wife, Carmela, as well.

Coach Scott Oatsvall (www.foodwars.org)

I want to first thank the Lord Jesus for rescuing my soul in 1989 and giving me His precious Holy Spirit.

A special thanks to my dear wife Carmela for being my constant channel for inspiration and encouragement. To Dave and Jan Dalton for inspiring me to embrace a healthy lifestyle and for introducing me to my co-author and brother from another mother, Coach Scott Oatsvall.

Finally, thank you to the board of Francis Myles International and my wonderful staff for working behind the scenes to make me and the ministry a success!

Dr. Francis Myles (www.foodwars.org)

FINDING
GOD
IN THE MIDDLE OF THE
FOOD
WARS

To live long and live well, we must be
healthy at the cellular level!

CONTENTS

FOREWORD

I T WAS 2013, AND I WAS SITTING IN A LARGE conference room in the Marriott Hotel, Brentwood, TN; there were about 75 people who, like me, were gathered to hear about healthy living. Coach Scott held the microphone with quiet confidence I had rarely seen in a speaker. After the meeting, I talked to someone who knew him and asked if they could tell me a little more about who he was. They immediately started to chuckle while shaking their head and gazing off to the side, almost like… there's a lot to say, where do I start! Then they just simply said, *"you aren't going to believe what he and his wife have done."* After he finished telling me, I was stunned. I remember walking away with my head shaking, looking down, and thinking, *"I have never known anyone with a resume of goodwill, selflessness, and philanthropy like this."* I didn't get to meet Coach Scott that day, but I didn't need to.

Coach Scott, who is never one to brag on himself, or what he had to overcome, was raised in the projects by a single mother. He carries no chip on his shoulder because of this fatherless misfortune. In fact, he embraces his past, which has become a major catalyst for his life. After high school, Coach Scott married his middle school sweetheart (Gwen). Yes, I said, middle school! Together, the two of them have become lifelong warriors (think of Jake Sully and Neytiri in the movie Avatar riding the great leonopteryx - red dragon). Both of them are truly defenders of the abandoned, abused, and forgotten children. Coach Scott and Gwen have two biological sons (Jeremiah and Elijah - two collegiate warriors in football), four adopted children, two from Uganda (Joseph and Daisy), and another two from China (Emily and Maggie), for a total of six.

Together they have partnered with community developments, schools, and homes for children in Uganda, Honduras, and Haiti. In addition, they provide food, clothing, school supplies, and essential items for 1000's at-risk and needy children in the Nashville area. Also, during this time, they served in a pastoral role in an inner-city church for several years.

Prior to their ministry, Coach Scott played division 1 football at San Diego State. He later went on to coach high school and then at the collegiate levels for 23 years.

In 2014 Coach Scott felt God calling him to the next chapter of his life, and he started a program called LT360 (Life Transformation 360); this was an outgrowth of his personal journey that nearly led to his early death, which he will tell you more about in the book. It was soon after this that I got to know him on a personal level. Coach Scott (along with Dr. Jae Hitson) co-founded one of Greater Nashville's most successful health clinics, LT360 Health Center. It is a functional medical and integrated health center with a full range of medical and holistic providers. In the past five years, they have helped 1000's of patients manage their weight, reverse chronic illnesses and disease while restoring themselves back to health. Coach Scott is like a mighty wind blowing into my sails. By the time you finish this book, I believe you will feel the same way!

Dr. Francis Myles and his lovely wife Carmela became a part of our lives a while back, but they have been guests at our home on several occasions. As a result, all of us have been fast-tracked on our friendship! I will never forget the first time I spoke with Dr. Myles, I was explaining our company and vision to him over the phone, and I was absolutely astonished at his ability to understand what we were doing. Normally, only those in the professional medical community can grasp the scope of our disruptive food technology (Wholeceuticals), but not Dr. Myles. He has a rare ability that I don't recall ever seeing in my life to grasp a wide range of academic and complex disciplines. It came as no surprise to me that Dr. Myles holds two doctoral degrees, but even that doesn't accurately measure his mental capacity.

Dr. Myles has authored many books, hosts a successful YouTube Channel (Francis Myles International) being watched by thousands every week. In addition to this, he holds conferences around the USA, and the world. We've had many discussions around food, and I noticed a remarkable connection Dr. Myles was able to make between food and the spirit world. As Christians, I think unless we see food for the spiritual role it can play in our life, we will by default succumb to its power to rule our appetite. The first book I read of his, "The Order of Melchizedek", which I believe will be a classic in the decades to come, felt like reading a modern-day Charles Spurgeon. I have read 100's of Christian books, no single book outside the Bible has had a more profound impact on me to this very day. As with me, Dr. Myles's ministry has been propelled forward by the support and inspiration from his gifted wife Carmela who carries a strong prophetic talent as a speaker and artist. I"m reminded every day when I put her beautifully designed prayer shawl over my head when I pray with my wife at our family altar.

I was "tapped on the shoulder" by Dr. Myles and Coach Scott to write this forward because of our food technology company, eBars. eBars mission is "to harness the full power of whole food." eBars has by "divine design" been operating, for the most part, in stealth for 9 years.

I have found through the years, that usually, the most life-changing events begin with a divine disruption. For some of you, this book will be a divine disruption. I encourage you to take a deep breath, and as a trusting child take the hand of Dr. Myles and Coach Scott and let them guide you to the place where you can live out your life the way God designed it to be.

God Bless Your Journey,

Dave Dalton
Founder: eBars

PREFACE

AT 27 YEARS OLD, I FOUND MYSELF ONE OF THE youngest head college coaches in the country. I had everything going for me, and the future looked bright...or did it?

You see, shortly after accepting that assignment, my health challenges started piling up: weight gain, high blood pressure, cholesterol issues, sleep disorders, and pre-diabetic, to name a few. "Wait a minute, that sounds like my grandparents. But I'm in my 20's!" For the next decade and a half, I battled health problems. I went on every weight loss program in America. I tried Weight Watchers, Jenny Craig, Adkins, every pill, powder, potion, and lotion to lose weight and get healthy. I went between 200 and almost 300 lbs. many times over the next ten years. At this time, I was on five medications. I was so discouraged and felt defeated. How could I be successful in so many areas of my public life and be a miserable failure in this private area?

After multiple emergency room visits in my early 40's, I had an event that would forever change my life. In March of 2011, at almost 300lbs, I thought I had a heart attack! I remember what my wife told me that day. She said, "Scott, you're going to die...and some other man is going to walk your daughters down the aisle!"

There are not words to describe that type of pain. The pain of regret is a pain that doesn't go away with a good night's sleep. At this point, I knew my life would change, but I wasn't sure how. So I have dedicated my life to help people get healthy at the cellular level, starting with me.

This book is the blueprint that God gave me to lose over 100lbs of fat and get off all medications. I have now been able to share the life-changing power of true transformation with thousands of my clients and patients. I pray that this framework will help you not only get healthy at the cellular level but find God in the process of becoming the best and highest version of you! Here's what it did for me.

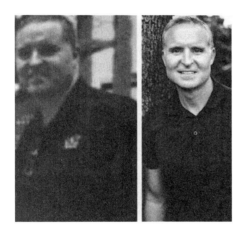

It's amazing to think of how our understanding of food and nutrition has grown in the past few decades related to our health and longevity. We call it Cellular Health. Using the principle that food is medicine will allow us to live healthy, happy, and whole lives for many years.

I live by the principle I call "SACC," which stands for Structure, Accountability, Coaching, and Community. By following these principles in both application and faith, we can keep our bodies healthy.

INTRODUCTION

L T360 HEALTH CENTER IS A FULLY INTEGRATED AND functional all- natural health care program. LT360 (Life Transformation 360) was founded in June of 2014 by Coach Scott Oatsvall.

Coach Scott was a high school teacher and college professor for 23 years. A health scare in his 40's forced him to re-evaluate his health. At the time, he was close to 300 pounds and on five medications – high blood pressure, high cholesterol, sleep apnea, Prilosec, and hypothyroidism.

Following a simple blueprint he had developed for himself, Coach Scott was off of all five of his medications in just six weeks. In a year, he lost 100 pounds of fat and has kept it off ever since. Family and friends began to ask for his help in finding the same freedom. Eventually, LT360 was born!

The mission of LT360 is to get you healthy at a cellular level and educate you in health, nutrition, fitness, motivation, and education. We provide individual coaching and motivate you every step of the way.

Our program gives you the structure, strategies, and support you need to reach your goals and transition to a healthier lifestyle, mind, body, and spirit. What started as a one-man operation is now a thriving, national business with thousands of clients in 29 states and nine foreign countries. For additional information about LT360 products, go to www.foodwars.org

TESTIMONIALS

"In 2016, I found myself desperate for answers to my weight gain and lack of energy despite many years of studying nutrition and working with doctors side-by-side teaching about nutrition.

In my mid-50's I heard about LT360 on the radio, and though I was highly skeptical, I had to learn more. I realized that Coach Scott Oatsvall had some missing pieces to my puzzle that could really make a difference. Applying the principles of LT360 has changed my life and given me more quality years. I am thrilled to say I went from a size 14 to a size four and gained back my energy, muscle tone, and great health. For nearly four years, I have had only one size in my closet, and I know everything will fit the same today as it has the past four years. At 61, I feel half my age. The structure, accountability, coaching, and community of LT360 made all the difference in the world! My medical doctor recently told me to save my money, that I will need it because I should live to be over 100!

You don't have to be an expert in nutrition to apply the principles of LT360! Anyone can do it, no matter what you enjoy eating, no matter how much or how little time you have, no matter what your health is at the time. LT360 meets you where you are and fits it into your lifestyle.

Now I am honored to be a Transformation Coach for LT360 for nearly two years. It gives me so much joy to watch people transform their lives and become their own health experts. They are like family to me.

I am so grateful for Scott Oatsvall, LT360, and the renewed health it has given me and so many others."

Elizabeth Murphy

❧❧

"August 9, 2016, was just another day in the life of a busy mom / daycare owner trying to find the energy and time to fit everything in her busy day. A friend of mine had tried to get me to go to an LT360 seminar for about four months, and some excuse always got in the way. Too expensive, too far to go to Franklin, kids got something to do, etc.

Being diagnosed as a Type 2 diabetic in November of 2015, losing 45lbs, then gaining 26 back, and continuing the yo-yo life, it was very appealing to me to think about losing weight and possibly getting off some meds, but honestly, I was very skeptical.

After hearing Coach Scott's testimony, I hit the ground running. After seven weeks on the program, I became disoriented at night, waking up, and sugar was bottoming out on me. I went to the doctor, and he took me off all medications! After seven weeks, diabetes meds, thyroid meds, restless leg, blood pressure, edema meds were removed!!! Praise the Lord

Now, almost 5-years later, no meds have been in my body!!! Not a Tylenol or a sinus pill. I feel amazing, and not only did my sick self become healed, but I also lost 110 lbs in 10 months and gained a community of LT360 family members that are so loving and supportive! I'm now a Coach on staff and have an office in my hometown in McMinnville, Tennessee, and a passion for helping change the lives of others like this program did mine. I'm a changed woman because of this program and my brother in Christ, Scott Oatsvall. A wonderful mentor and friend for whom I thank my God daily."

Tammy McDonald Young

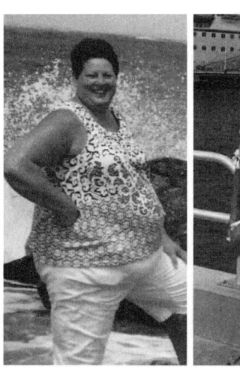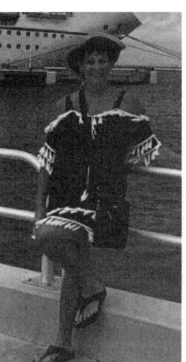

SECTION ONE

BIBLICAL PATHOLOGIES BEHIND
FOOD ADDICTION
AND SPIRITUAL WELL BEING

Dr. Francis Myles

Therefore, I urge you, brothers and sisters, in view of God's mercy, to offer your bodies as a living sacrifice, holy and pleasing to God--this is your true and proper worship.

Romans 12:1 NLT

1

IT ALL BEGAN WITH ONE BITE!

Then the LORD God took the man and put him in the garden of Eden to tend and keep it. ¹⁶ And the LORD God commanded the man, saying, "Of every tree of the garden you may freely eat; ¹⁷ but of the tree of the knowledge of good and evil you shall not eat, for in the day that you eat of it you[f] shall surely die."

Genesis 2:15-17

I WANT TO BEGIN THIS CHAPTER BY POSING VERY fundamental and philosophical questions; "Does eating matter?" More importantly, "Does what you eat matter?" One would think the answer to the first question is obvious. However, most answers to this question will be purely biological and sociological as many people in this world "live to eat" instead of "eating to live." There is a vast difference between these two ideologies. The latter is by divine design, whereas the former is due to foods designed to be addictive, engineered by a corrupt, profit-driven food industry. My co-author, Coach Scott Oatsvall, a highly esteemed health and wellness coach to thousands of clients, will go into greater detail unmasking the food industry's dangerous lies. It's an open secret that many key players in the food space prioritize quick profits over its consumers' general and physical well-being. *The truth is, the kitchen table kills more people every year than many of us can imagine.*

This leads us back to my second question, "Does what you eat matter?" More than the first, this question is the primary reason Coach Scott and I wrote this book. Whether you know it or not, there is a "global war" raging all over the world over which food or foods penetrate your mouth. Since eating is essential to man's physical survival and well-being, food is the most significant industry on earth. Companies and food scientists are determined to control this very lucrative global market at whatever cost. That is why multinational pharmaceutical corporations are heavily invested in creating "GMO foods (Genetically Modified Organism)." Unfortunately, they are flooding grocery stores worldwide with GMO foods that many of which God never intended for us to eat. As the name suggests, GMO food is food from a seed whose original, God-given genetic properties have been tampered with to create a *food seed* that can be patented as a corporation's intellectual property. Is it then surprising that many of these genetically modified foods have the power to alter our God- given DNA when consumed continuously over time??

THE FORBIDDEN FRUIT

"But of the tree of the knowledge of good and evil you shall not eat, for in the day that you eat of it, you shall surely die."

—Genesis 2:17

One of my favorite books in the Bible is the book of Genesis. God's original intent for His creation is also hidden within the pages of this book. It is no wonder it is called the book of beginnings or "Bereshit" in the Hebrew language. Please remember, *things don't end wrong; they start wrong.* That is why God is very concerned about the beginning of a thing. To understand the power of eating or the power of food in general, we need to go back to the Garden of Eden. God-approved eating (i.e., healthy eating) began in this glorious garden of abundance. Unfortunately, satanically engineered eating (unhealthy and death-causing eating) also sprang from the same garden. The first man and woman on earth, Adam and Eve, were the first people to eat the food, God created. Unfortunately, Adam and Eve are also responsible for opening the door for the entrance of satanically engineered (altered), death-causing foods into the world of men.

God never hid the fact that all eating is not equal. He warned Adam and Eve, most especially Adam, who was created first, that he could eat of every tree in the garden, but he could not eat of the tree of the "Knowledge of Good and Evil." The penalty for violating this divine instruction would be both spiritual and physical death. The moral of the story; God was telling Adam that there's a modality of eating that opens the door for the technology of death to invade the human experience. Since eating is also a spiritual act of worship towards God, there is a "way of eating" that desensitizes man's spirit from effectively interacting with God. That means there is a way of eating that empowers Satan to take control of the human body as a vehicle for advancing his demonic agenda here on earth at the expense of God's original intent for creating man's humus body. However, before we explore in detail the entrance of satanically engineered, death-causing foods, it behooves us to first understand man's original God-given diet.

LIFE-GIVING FOOD!

So God said, "Behold, I have given you every plant yielding seed that is on the surface of the entire earth, and every tree which has fruit yielding seed; it shall be food for you; ³⁰ and to all the animals on the earth and to every bird of the air and to everything that moves on the ground—to everything in which there is the breath of life—I have given every green plant for food"; and it was so [because He commanded it]. ³¹ God saw everything that He had made, and behold, it was very good, and He validated it completely.

—Genesis 1:29-31 (AMP)

God's highest currency is life. No one can give life except God. Thus, life is God's highest gift to man. It amazes me that even with our technological and scientific advancements, we have not figured out how to recreate life! It's not just human life that we have failed to re-create; we have failed to re-create the life of the simplest lifeforms on earth. If we kill a bug or a deer, there exists no human technology or medical device that can recreate the life of that specific bug or deer. However, in the typical arrogance of our fallen nature, even though we cannot re-create life, we have no reservations about killing it, whether through government- sanctioned abortions or the gradual dying process which is induced by wrongful eating.

From the above passage of scripture, it is clear that God's original intent and diet for the optimal performance of man's body was the eating of *"every plant yielding seed that is on the surface of the entire earth and every tree which has fruit yielding seed."* In other words, Adam and Eve and all wildlife were vegetarians before the fall of man in the Garden of Eden. If Adam and Eve had not fallen into sin and bite into the devil's lie, both mankind and wild animals would never have known the taste of meat. I am not suggesting in any way that the readers of this book become vegetarians. Post-Garden of Eden, God, in His eternal genius and mercy toward mankind, expanded our dietary menu to include meat and other healthy foods that are not fruits and vegetables. However, some of the healthiest people I have met are vegetarians. My co-author, Coach Scott Oatsvall, will guide us through an expanded list of life-giving foods that go beyond fruits and vegetables. These foods will help you lose weight and become healthy at the cellular level while helping your body regenerate itself!

> Then the angel showed me a river of the water of life, clear as crystal, flowing from the throne of God and of the Lamb (Christ), ² in the middle of its street. On either side of the river was the tree of life, bearing twelve kinds of fruit, yielding its fruit every month; and the leaves of the tree were for the healing of the nations.
>
> —Revelation 22:1-2

The book of Genesis is the book of beginnings, while the book of Revelation is a book of endings; it is the book that shows us how God corrects what was broken in the beginning. So, it is not surprising that the last chapter in the book of Revelation has to do with the restoration of man's original diet, which we now discover is actually a heavenly diet. It is the Apostle John who is shown a powerful vision of *"a river of the water of life, clear as crystal, flowing from the throne of God, on either side of the river was the tree of life, bearing twelve kinds of fruit, yielding its fruit every month; and the leaves of the tree were for the healing of the nations."* In the end, mankind will return to the original diet God gave to Adam and Eve in the Garden of Eden. A diet of fruits and vegetables, with the "leaves" being for the healing of the nations. The expression in the scriptural passage, *"the leaves of the tree were for the healing of the nations"* is meant to convey the idea that **true life-giving food is also supposed to act as a medicine to the human body.** This divine plumbline is what Coach Scott Oatsvall will discuss throughout this book. He will show you which foods act as medicine to the human body for optimal performance at the cellular level. He will also show you foods (many of you enjoy) that act as poisons in your temple (body).

THE BEGINNING OF DEATH-CAUSING EATING!

> Now the serpent was more cunning than any beast of the field which the LORD God had made. And he said to the woman, "Has God indeed said, 'You shall not eat of every tree of the garden'?" ² And the woman said to the serpent, "We may eat the fruit of the trees of the garden; ³ but of the fruit of the tree which is in the midst of the garden, God has said, 'You shall not eat it, nor shall you touch it, lest you die.'" ⁴ Then the serpent said to the woman, "You will not surely die. ⁵ For God knows that in the day you eat of it your eyes will be opened, and you will be like God, knowing good and evil." ⁶ So when the woman saw that the tree was good for food, that it was pleasant to the eyes, and a tree desirable to make one wise, she took of its fruit and ate. She also gave to her husband with her, and he ate. ⁷ Then the eyes of both of them were opened, and they knew that they were naked; and they sewed fig leaves together and made themselves coverings.
>
> —Genesis 3:1-7

How did it all start? How did eating open the door of death? I will never forget where I was in 2006 when the "King of Pop," Michael Jackson, died. I was preaching at one of my favorite churches in

Bloomfield, Connecticut, when I received the news. Millions of Michael Jackson fans worldwide went into a period of intense mourning for this legendary music icon. In the postmortem, it was discovered that he had died from an overdose of sleeping pills prescribed to him by his doctor. So, the cause of death was not in question. What would you say if I told you that the *silver bullet of death* which struck Michael Jackson could be traced back to a seemingly innocent conversation thousands of years ago? A conversation in a garden between Eve and a malicious serpent convinced her that "eating of the fruit" of the forbidden tree would have no deadly consequences. Would you believe me? Some of you might be tempted to say I'm stretching the truth. But am I? If Adam and Eve had not eaten of the tree of the knowledge of good and evil, would we be experiencing death? If the answer is "No," then the legendary Michael Jackson was not killed by sleeping pills. But he was killed by the same technology of death which Satan unleashed into the world of men by convincing the first couple that "all-eating," including that which God has forbidden, is equal!

In the above scripture, Satan, masquerading as a talking serpent in the Garden of Eden, initiated a conversation with Eve. The conversation was designed to question an instruction that God had given them concerning what they could and could not eat. In Satan's typical deceptive fashion, he feigned ignorance about what kind of eating God had restricted, by generalizing his question, *"Has God indeed said, 'You shall not eat of every tree of the garden'?"* However, Satan's true intention was to open up a conversation with an unsuspecting woman to sow doubts about the only tree from which Adam and Eve were not allowed to eat, *the tree of the Knowledge Of Good And Evil.*

Satan planned to introduce mankind to "death-causing eating" or "appetites" that inevitably lead to him gaining more control over man's spirit, soul, and body! All he needed to gain a legal foothold over the world of men and take over is **"just one bite"** of the fruit from the forbidden tree! Let the power of that statement sink into your spirit as you meditate on its far-reaching implications! All the turmoil on earth, all the stealing, all the suffering, and all the dying that we see today **began with just one bite!** This would certainly not be possible if eating food was not both a spiritual and physical act. Understanding the fact that "eating is first and foremost spiritual" before its natural is the divine plumbline that weaves its way throughout this book from the first to the last chapter. We must remember that man is a "spirit being" having a bodily experience. Consequently deciding to "lose weight" as a result of any diet will mostly likely end in failure if the decision to lose weight and get healthy is void of a more compelling spiritual reason. God indeed wants us to eat and enjoy what we eat! However, God does not want us to poison our bodies eating junk food! New Testament scripture is clear; our bodies have been bought with the price of the blood of Jesus, and we are now the temple of the Holy Spirit. Consequently, what we put inside our temple (body) is very important to God both as a spiritual and practical matter. Amen.

LIFE APPLICATION SECTION

Memory Verse

Whose fate is destruction, whose god is their belly [their worldly appetite, their sensuality, their vanity], and whose glory is in their shame—who focus their mind on earthly and temporal things.

—Philippians 3:19

Reflections

1. What is the name of the tree that God told Adam and Eve not to eat its fruit?

_____

_____

_____

_____

2. How did Satan manipulate our desire to eat to become the god of this world?

_____

_____

_____

_____

2

JACOB HAVE I LOVED, BUT ESAU HAVE I HATED!

As it is written, "Jacob I have loved, but Esau I have hated."

Romans 9:13

WHEN I FIRST CAME ACROSS THE ABOVE PASSAGE of scripture, I was totally baffled by it! Knowing God's character as one who is full of unconditional love and acceptance for His creation, it was a difficult pill for me to swallow, theologically speaking. Please remember that this passage of scripture was declared by God long before Jacob and Esau were born, which then causes one to ponder why God loved one child while hating the other when He created them both? That was my dilemma until the Holy Spirit gave me the hidden revelation or meaning behind this verse. When I finally saw it, I worshiped God for His infinite wisdom. I also came into some understanding about how serious God treats our natural appetites. It is this revelation that prepared me to co-author this book with Coach Scott Oatsvall. I will spend this entire chapter unpacking this amazing revelation. However, I want to first unpack the prophetic events which surrounded the birth of these unlikely twins.

TWO NATIONS ARE IN YOUR WOMB

> Now Isaac pleaded with the LORD for his wife, because she was barren: and the and the LORD granted his plea, and Rebekah his wife conceived. ²² But the children struggled together within her; and she said, "If all is well, why am I like this?" So she went to inquire of the LORD.²³ And the LORD said to her: "Two nations are in your womb, Two peoples shall be separated from your body; One people shall be stronger than the other, And the older shall serve the younger."
>
> —Genesis 25:21-23

Esau and Jacob's birth was due to God's divine intervention in response to Isaac's prayer for his barren wife, Rebecca. She had not been able to conceive for quite some time. God answered the prayer of Isaac for his beloved wife, and she became pregnant with twins. As her pregnancy reached a maturation stage, the children began to wrestle against each other within her womb. This created severe physical and emotional discomfort for Rebecca. She ran to God and asked Him why there was so much turmoil in her womb. God responded by telling her, *"Two nations are in your womb, two peoples shall be separated from your body; One people shall be stronger than the other, and the older shall serve the younger."* God's perspective of things is truly different from ours.

God always keeps in mind the bigger picture! If Rebecca had asked any of us, we would've said she was pregnant with two babies, but none of us would have said she was pregnant with two nations! However, since it's God who said it, we have to believe that Rebecca's twins represent two types of nations of people here on earth.

Therefore, it behooves us to understand the divine plumbline line that separates these two nations of people.

To discover this divine plumbline, we must tiptoe around the lives of these two boys to discover what spiritual element became the most distinctive difference between them. In following Esau's life, it becomes pretty evident that his life lacked any obvious passion for God. He was a hunter of wild animals with an outgoing outdoor personality. There is no scripture reference of Esau praying to God or having any extraordinary encounter with God. On the other hand, Jacob stayed very close to his mother, Rebecca, who nurtured his passion for God by rehearsing in his ears the prophecy God gave her concerning the nature of his birth and destiny. The prophecy created in him a deep desire to know God intimately. However, in his untrained spiritual eye, Jacob felt like his brother's firstborn birthright would get in the way of him receiving God's best. So, he concocted a plan to compel his elder brother to sell his God-given birthright!

BIRTHRIGHT FOR A BOWL OF SOUP

Jacob had cooked [reddish-brown lentil] stew [one day], when Esau came from the field and was famished; ³⁰ and Esau said to Jacob, "Please, let me have a quick swallow of that red stuff there because I am exhausted and famished." For that reason, Esau was [also] called Edom (Red). ³¹ Jacob answered, "First sell me your birthright (the rights of a firstborn)." ³² Esau said, "Look, I am about to die [if I do not eat soon]; so, of what use is this birthright to me?" ³³ Jacob said, "Swear [an oath] to me today [that you are selling it to me for this food]"; so, he swore [an oath] to him and sold him his birthright. ³⁴ Then Jacob gave Esau bread and

32

lentil stew; and he ate and drank and got up and went on his way. In this way, Esau scorned his birthright.

—Genesis 25:29-34

Fortunately, we did not have to wait long to discover the critical difference, that spiritual element, that distinguished Jacob from Esau for the rest of their life. Since Jacob spent a lot of time with his mother in the kitchen, he became very proficient at cooking. According to the above passage of scripture, in the course of time, there came a day when Esau came from the field hungry and desired to eat right away. Sensing that this was his opportunity to capture his brother's firstborn birthright, Jacob took a chance at negotiating the deal of the century.

THE FIRSTBORN BLESSING!

"You shall not delay the offering from your harvest and your vintage. You shall give (consecrate, dedicate) to Me the firstborn of your sons. ³⁰ You shall do the same with your oxen and with your sheep. It shall be with its mother for seven days; on the eighth day, you shall give it [as an offering] to Me.

—Exodus 22:29-30

At the beginning of this chapter, I told you how Romans 9:13 bothered me theologically for a very long time. But one day, when I was reading the Bible, the Holy Spirit finally unveiled the mystery of this statement. In the ancient world's Hebraic Semitic tradition, there was nothing more precious, sacred, and invaluable as being the firstborn son. The firstborn son was responsible for carrying on the family name and father's legacy. Most importantly, the first-born son was responsible for carrying the revelation of the father's God to the next generation. In essence, being the firstborn son was a priestly position. In the Old Testament, the firstborn son was the one who typically received a double inheritance and was the one who would inherit his father's role as head of the family. It is no wonder God used the death of the first-born son to break the back of Egypt, forcing Pharaoh to let the children of Israel go finally! Exodus 12:29-30 declares, *"Now it happened at midnight that the LORD struck every firstborn in the land of Egypt, from the firstborn of Pharaoh who sat on his throne to the firstborn of the prisoner who was in the [a]dungeon, and all the firstborn of the cattle. ³⁰ Pharaoh got up in the night, he and all his servants and all the Egyptians, and there was a great cry [of heartache and sorrow] in Egypt, for there was no house where there was not someone dead."* The emotional blow of losing their firstborn sons was too much for the Egyptians to handle. They lifted their hands and surrendered to God. Even though they were heathens who worshiped countless idols, they knew the importance and sacredness of the firstborn son.

> He is the exact living image [the essential manifestation] of the unseen God [the visible representation of the invisible], the firstborn [the preeminent one, the sovereign, and the originator] of all creation.
> —Colossians 1:15

The term firstborn has two meanings. The first is more literal, referring to the fact that this son is the first son to be born of his father. The second meaning refers to the rights, privileges, and authority of a person simply because they are the firstborn. According to Colossians 1:15, Jesus is the firstborn in several ways, as the most pre-imminent being in all of creation. Most importantly, Jesus' position as the "firstborn of all creation and the firstborn from the dead" means that He is the one God has appointed to be in authority over all things in heaven, earth, and under the earth! Since the Old Testament is a revelation of Jesus, it suddenly makes sense. In the book of Exodus, God made it very clear that the firstborn of both man and animal belonged to the Lord: this was a special blessing and assignment that was only given to the firstborn son. You may be wondering why I'm spending so much time talking about the blessing of the firstborn son in a book about *Finding God in the Middle of the Food Wars*. That's a fair question, which leads us to the next paragraph and a climactic revelation of this entire book's essence.

JACOB HAVE I LOVED, BUT ESAU HAVE I HATED!

As it is written, "Jacob I have loved, but Esau have I hated."
—Romans 9:13

Now that you appreciate the sacredness and importance of the blessing of the firstborn son within the canon of Scripture, we will examine the far-reaching spiritual implications of what transpired between Esau and Jacob involving a cup of soup. With forensic aptitude, let us now examine the conversation between the two brothers and the deal that they struck that triggered irreversible consequences in Esau's life in both heaven and earth. I will add my comments to each statement of the conservation so you don't lose the essence of what transpired between the two brothers that caused God to say, *"Jacob have I loved, Esau have I hated."*

Esau said to Jacob, "Please, let me have a quick swallow of that red stuff there, because I am exhausted and famished." There is nothing wrong with being hungry or famished. It's natural, normal, and healthy to recognize when your body is telling you to eat. However, how you go about satisfying your legitimate hunger says a lot about you and what's whole or broken inside of you.

Jacob answered, "First sell me your birthright (the rights of a firstborn)." This should've been the end of the discussion. I've already shown you how sacred and priceless position the firstborn son was to both his natural father and to Father God Almighty. If I were Esau, I would've rebuked my young brother for even suggesting such a thing, let alone contemplate it with any seriousness. The suggestion was ridiculous and unreasonable. The priceless nature of the rights of the firstborn far outweighed any benefit, physical or spiritual, that could be gained from consuming one bowl of soup.

Nevertheless, how did Esau respond? Esau said, *"Look, I am about to die [if I do not eat soon];* This is Satan's classic lie that if you don't eat right away, you are going to die! Coach Scott and many natural path doctors will tell you that it's biologically impossible for the human body to enter the realm of "true hunger" within 24 hours! An article in the National Library of Medicine states the body can survive for 8 to 21 days without food and water and up to two months if there's access to an adequate water intake. Modern-day hunger strikes have provided insight into starvation. One study in the *British Medical Journal Trusted Source* cited several hunger strikes that ended after 21 to 40 days." Coach Scott Oatsvall will show you that much of the "false- hunger" our body experiences is due to eating foods that are not healthy but are designed to entice us to eat more than we should!

"So, of what use is this birthright to me?" I want you to digest the level of arrogance and spiritual apathy that is contained in this one statement. Esau saw the sacred gift of being the firstborn son as a thing so trivial he did not see how it could benefit him when he was hungry and just wanted to eat right away! So, he quickly despised the priceless gift of being the firstborn son without even thinking about it! This was the equivalent of pointing a finger in God's face. And for what? Just to gulp down a bowl of soup! It was tragic, to say the least.

Jacob said, "Swear [an oath] to me today [that you are selling it to me for this food]." More than anything else, it was this oath that was the reason God says, "Esau I hate, and Jacob have I loved." By asking him to swear, Jacob was giving Esau the opportunity to appreciate the gravity and irreversibility of the transaction before them. Jacob made it clear that if Esau took the cup of soup and drunk from it, he was selling his God-given rights as the firstborn son in exchange for food! It was the worst business proposition a Semitic person of that era could have been given.

IT'S THE SPIRIT BEHIND ESAU THAT GOD HATES!

> So, he swore [an oath] to him, and sold him his birthright.
> ³⁴ Then Jacob gave Esau bread and lentil stew; and he ate and drank and got up and went on his way. In this way Esau scorned his birthright.
> —Genesis 25:33-34

After the Holy Spirit unpacked the revelation and the mystery behind the statement, "Esau I hate and Jacob have I loved," He said to me; "Francis, it's not Esau the man that I hated, it's the spirit in him that says food is more important than matters of destiny. I hate the demonic spirit that causes my people to choose food over their God-given birthright." A lightbulb of understanding flipped on inside of me, and I finally saw it! Suddenly, Romans 9:13 was no longer a theological dilemma for me. I finally understood what God was saying. Since then, I've come across preachers of the gospel who will not even take one day to fast! They are so addicted to food! Their idea of fasting is not watching TV for a couple of hours, but don't you dare touch the food on their plate! They will attack you like a pack of hyenas. Esau swore an oath to his brother and sold him his birthright in exchange for food. Jacob wasted no time consummating the deal of the century. He quickly gave Esau bread and lentil stew; Esau ate, drank, and then went on his way. Sadly, for a piece of bread and some lentil stew, Esau scorned his God-given birthright as the first-born son. Since the transaction was legal, heaven, earth, and hell all recognized it. Years later, when Esau finally realized the far-reaching spiritual implications of what he had done, he tried to reverse course, but to no avail! The writer of the book of Hebrews records it this way!

> And [see to it] that no one is immoral or godless like Esau, who sold his own birthright for a single meal. ¹⁷ For you know that later on, when he wanted [to regain title to] his inheritance of the blessing, he was rejected, for he found no opportunity for repentance [there was no way to repair what he had done, no chance to recall the choice he had made], even though he sought for it with [bitter] tears.
>
> —Hebrews 12:16-17

LIFE, DESTINY, OR FRIED CHICKEN!

When my wife and I were pastoring our first church in Arizona, I came face-to-face with the outworking of this satanic principle that operated in Esau. A couple who loved our ministry moved from one of the Midwestern states to join our church and ministry in Phoenix, Arizona. My wife and I were delighted to have this couple join us because we knew them before moving to Arizona to plant a church. They quickly submerged themselves into the ministry and began to form very strong friendships within the church. One Sunday, I was engrossed in preaching when one of our clinically trained ushers noticed Mrs. Polly (not her real name) was having difficulty breathing. The usher called 911, and they sent an ambulance to take Sister Polly to the hospital. When service was over, I inquired about what had transpired.

My wife and I rushed to the hospital to check up on her! She was in good spirits. Her husband was sitting next to her hospital bed. However, the doctor gave her a stern warning. Mrs. Polly was told that her arteries were very clogged due to many years of eating deep-fried foods in the southern cooking style in which she was raised. The doctor warned her against continuing to eat these fried foods. Her arteries were so bad the doctor told her not to eat fried chicken, period!

While she was with the doctor, she agreed with him, but as soon as she was discharged, she simply laughed it off! In her mind, the doctor was being overly cautious. There was no way she was going to give up eating her favorite fried chicken dish at her age! Her husband argued with her and begged her to listen to the doctor's orders. But she wouldn't have it any other way! One day she decided to cook her favorite fried chicken dinner. Later, her husband told me that they had argued about her cooking that meal. Unfortunately, she prevailed! Mrs. Polly ate her favorite fried chicken dinner, which became her last meal here on earth. It was not long before she was again rushed to the hospital because she had a heart attack! By the time the ambulance got to the hospital, there was nothing the doctors could do for her. She was already dead! Even though she loved the Lord, she forfeited her God-given destiny because she would not let go of her fried chicken dinner. It is then Romans 9:13 went even deeper inside of me. I came to fully appreciate what God meant when He said, **"Jacob have I loved, but Esau have I hated."** God hates with a passion that spirit that causes His people to choose food over their priceless God-given destiny! If only the graveyard could talk, it would tell us of multiplied thousands of men and women who died before their appointed time because they couldn't let go of their so-called "favorite foods" that were killing them slowly!

LIFE APPLICATION SECTION

Memory Verse

And [see to it] that no one is immoral or godless like Esau, who sold his own birthright for a single meal. ¹⁷ For you know that later on, when he wanted [to regain title to] his inheritance of the blessing, he was rejected, for he found no opportunity for repentance [there was no way to repair what he had done, no chance to recall the choice he had made], even though he sought for it with [bitter] tears.

—Hebrews 12:16-17

Reflections

1. For what did Esau trade his firstborn birthright?

_____

_____

_____

_____

2. What does the expression, "Jacob have I loved, but Esau have I hated" mean?

_____

_____

_____

_____

Therefore I consider all your precepts
to be right; I hate every false way.

Psalm 119:128 ESV

3

THE SPIRITUALITY OF DIET

So then, whether you eat or drink or whatever you do, do all to the glory of [our great] God.

1 Corinthians 10:31

THE ABOVE PASSAGE OF SCRIPTURE MAKES IT abundantly clear that eating and drinking are spiritual. Eating and drinking are not just natural exercises, and therefore the Apostle Paul admonishes believers to conform both their eating and drinking to the glory of God. Coach Scott Oatsvall's contribution to this book will clearly show why Paul wrote the above scripture passage. Coach will make it very clear that what we eat or drink can either extend our lifespan or shorten it. This statement begs the question, "if life is a gift from God, then doesn't it follow that we owe it to God to steward our temple (our body) in the most cautious way possible?" Have you been to a funeral lately and seen the finality of death: the tears and lamentations of regret that family members and friends of the deceased pour over the coffin of the dearly departed? I am convinced that if most of the dead got an opportunity to attend their own funerals and see the emotional devastation their premature departure inflicted on their loved ones, many would've made better choices concerning the food they ate or the drinks they drank.

IT WAS A SET-UP!

And the [Babylonian] king told Ashpenaz, the chief of his [d]officials, to bring in some of the sons of Israel, including some from the royal family and from the nobles, ⁴ young men without blemish and handsome in appearance, skillful in all wisdom, endowed with intelligence and discernment, and quick to understand, competent to stand [in the presence of the king] and able to serve in the king's palace. He also ordered Ashpenaz to teach them the literature and language of the Chaldeans the Chaldeans. ⁵ The king assigned a daily ration for them from his finest food and from the wine which he drank. They were to be educated and nourished this way for three years so that at the end of that time they were [prepared] to enter the king's service. ⁶ Among them from the sons of Judah were: Daniel, Hananiah, Mishael, and Azariah.

—Daniel 1:3-6

The book of Daniel begins by describing the destruction of Jerusalem by the Babylonian king known as King Nebuchadnezzar. King Nebuchadnezzar was allowed by God to take some of the holiest articles from the temple of God in Jerusalem to Babylon. In his conquest, King Nebuchadnezzar also captured several Hebrew boys from Jewish houses of nobility. He wanted to train them in the ways of the Babylonians so that they could work within his palace. One of those Hebrew boys was Daniel, who was accompanied by three others, Hananiah, Mishael, and Azariah. If one were looking at the circumstances that these four Hebrew boys found themselves in, one would be tempted to say they were victims of their circumstances and not champions of the own destinies. However, nothing could be further from the truth when you examine how the events in the book of Daniel panned out. If you examine the entire book of Daniel, you discover that it was about the clash of kingdoms, most notably the clash between the Kingdom of Light versus the kingdom of darkness. In every instance in the book of Daniel where there was a face-to-face clash of kingdoms, the Kingdom of Light took the crown! Once, the Lord showed me that He did not take Daniel and the other three Hebrew boys to Babylon to have them live in captivity. Actually, in God's creative genius, God allowed King Nebuchadnezzar to capture them so that He could use them to demonstrate the superiority of the gospel of the Kingdom of God in a culture that provided such a stark contrast with God's. In other words, Daniel's capture was a divine setup!

Interestingly enough, the first clash of kingdoms in Babylon was over diet, that is, food. It is very revealing that the first battle in this clash of kingdoms was over which kingdom had a superior, life-enhancing diet for its citizens! A battle that God won decisively!

DANIEL PURPOSED IN HIS HEART!

But Daniel purposed in his heart that he would not defile himself with the portion of the king's delicacies, nor with the wine which he drank; therefore, he requested of the chief of the eunuchs that he might not defile himself. 9 Now God had brought Daniel into the favor and goodwill of the chief of the eunuchs. 10 And the chief of the eunuchs said to Daniel, "I fear my lord the king, who has appointed your food and drink. For why should he see your faces looking

* worse than the young men who are your age? Then you would endanger my head before the king."

—Daniel 1:8-10

The story of Daniel takes a sudden turn when Daniel and his three Hebrew counterparts purpose in their heart they would not defile themselves with the portion of the king's delicacies, nor with the wine which he drank. This was borderline insulting at best or treasonous at worst. King Nebuchadnezzar's chief eunuch was appalled and perplexed by Daniel's decision. Who in their right mind refuses to eat from the king's table adorned with delicate dishes from every part of the kingdom? The Babylonian king was reputed to have some of the best chefs from around the world. The wine that was served at his meals were vintage wines from the best vineyards in Babylon. Any lessor human would've killed to be invited to the king's table, but Daniel was not impressed.

Daniel, Hananiah, Mishael, and Azariah, knew that the Babylonians were notorious for dedicating their food to the altars of the demon gods that they worshiped. In some cases, some of the Babylonian delicacies were mixed with the blood of animals or humans who were sacrificed at the altars of these demon gods. Even though Daniel was a man of intense prayer, he realized that praying over the food on the king's table would not have been as effective as abstaining from eating these foods altogether. I guess Daniel was sending New Testament Christians a message, no amount of praying can truly insulate us from the side-effects of genetically compromised food. Most Christians use prayer to justify eating some of the most toxic foods on the planet: a sad truth revealed by the growing number of premature deaths in the Body of Christ! However, some prayers are not necessary if we dare use common sense and wisdom. It is not unspiritual or a sign of unbelief to read the ingredients in food in the grocery store before buying, cooking, and eating it. The FDA (Food & Drug Administration) has done its part to force the food industry to label all the ingredients they use to make certain foods so that consumers can make healthy choices as to what they eat or not! So, please do your part and take time to read the ingredients in the foods you eat. You'll be shocked to discover that some of your favorite foods are the worst foods you can ever put in your temple (body). Selah!

PUT IT TO A TEST!

> So Daniel said to the steward whom the chief of the eunuchs had set over Daniel, Hananiah, Mishael, and Azariah, ¹² "Please test your servants for ten days, and let them give us vegetables to eat and water to drink. ¹³ Then let our appearance be examined before you, and the appearance of the young men who eat the portion of the king's delicacies; and as you see fit, so deal with your servants." ¹⁴ So he consented with them in this matter and tested them ten days.
>
> —Daniel 1:11-14

The steward whom the chief of the eunuchs had set over Daniel, Hananiah, Mishael, and Azariah, was deathly terrified that if Daniel and his counterparts did not fare as well as the others who were eating the king's delicacies his head would be on the chopping block. Daniel, brimming with confidence over the opportunity to demonstrate the superiority of "food by God," assured the steward that nothing worse would happen to them. However, to ease the conscience of the steward, Daniel proposed a simple but effective test! The test that he proposed could only come from somebody who absolute confidence in the effectiveness of the diet he was proposing. Daniel said, *"Please test your servants for ten days, and let them give us vegetables to eat and water to drink. Then let our appearance be examined before you, and the appearance of the young men who eat the portion of the king's delicacies; and as you see fit, so deal with your servants."*

King Nebuchadnezzar's steward, who was over Daniel and his friends, relaxed at the proposal. He knew that ten days was not such a long time that he could not reverse his decision and save his neck if the whole experiment turned out to be a total disaster. Nevertheless, he was not aware of the utter shock he would be experiencing at the complete superiority of Daniel's divinely inspired diet. At the end of the agreed-upon ten days, Daniel, Hananiah, Mishael, and Azariah's healthy appearance was breathe taking! Their countenance was like that of an angel! The steward of King Nebuchadnezzar had never seen anything like it in his life!

The problem with most Christians is that they are so addicted to wrong and genetically modified foods that they have lost the taste for the life-giving *"food by God."* As you are reading this book, I double dare you to do what Daniel did and put *"food by God"* to the test, then see what happens to your health, vitality, and spiritual well-being!

FOOD BY GOD WINS!

> And at the end of ten days their features appeared better and fatter in flesh than all the young men who ate the portion of the king's delicacies. [16] Thus the steward took away their portion of delicacies and the wine that they were to drink and gave them vegetables.
>
> —Daniel 1:15-16

What was the *"food by God"* that Daniel suggested to the steward to become their daily diet for ten days? It was water and vegetables; this means that during the 10-day diet testing period, Daniel, Hananiah,

Mishael, and Azariah, ate no red meat or any other animal fat. They were on a strict vegetarian diet. They had essentially gone back to the beginning. Genesis 1:29 says, *"So God said, "Behold, I have given you every plant yielding seed that is on the surface of the entire earth, and every tree which has fruit yielding seed; it shall be food for you."* I am in no way suggesting that Daniel and his three Hebrew friends lived on vegetables and water for the remainder of the 70 years they were in Babylon. If you're confused on which foods to eat that fall under the category of *"food by God,"* you will never go wrong eating vegetables and fruits. That said, the New Testament shows us that the Lord Jesus Christ ate meat, fish, and vegetables, and He even ate unleavened bread. Jesus also drank wine. The greatest prophet of them all, John the Baptist, ate wild locust and honey. That shows us that there are various *"foods by God"* that we can eat which will not compromise our physical health and spiritual vitality.

10 TIMES BETTER!

Now at the end of the days, when the king had said that they should be brought in, the chief of the eunuchs brought them in before Nebuchadnezzar. ¹⁹ Then the king interviewed them, and among them all none was found like Daniel, Hananiah, Mishael, and Azariah; therefore, they served before the king. ²⁰ And in all matters of wisdom and understanding about which the king examined them, he found them ten times better than all the magicians and astrologers who were in all his realm.

—Daniel 1:18-20

Something shockingly supernatural and life-changing happened at the end of King Nebuchadnezzar's training for all the nobles' children. The chief of the eunuchs brought the graduating class before King Nebuchadnezzar. When the king started interviewing them, he found none like Daniel, Hananiah, Mishael, and Azariah. According to the above scripture, *"in all matters of wisdom and understanding about which the king examined them, he found them **ten times** better than all the magicians and astrologers who were in all his realm."* I want you to let the implications of this statement sink into your spirit!

In everything King Nebuchadnezzar tested them on, the four Hebrew boys who had been living on the diet of *"food by God,"* he discovered that their mental acuteness was off the charts! Their IQ was ten times better in every subject of governance, science, astrology, and even Babylonian culture. For those of us who have bought into the lie that what you eat and drink does not affect our intelligence, the story of Daniel and the three Hebrew boys should give serious pause. Could it be that the lack of intelligence that is becoming almost a pandemic in the Body of Christ results from the foods we eat? Many of the foods we are eating are making us mentally dull and spiritually lazy. I am very convinced that by the time you finish reading this book, you will never again take the issue of food very lightly. For most of you, you will be well on your way to recovering your God-given health, accompanied by the weight loss that you have been seeking all your life!

LIFE APPLICATION SECTION

Memory Verse

"Please test your servants for ten days and let them give us vegetables to eat and water to drink. ¹³ Then let our appearance be examined before you, and the appearance of the young men who eat the portion of the king's delicacies; and as you see fit, so deal with your servants." ¹⁴ So he consented with them in this matter and tested them ten days.

—Daniel 1:12-14

Reflections

1. What diet did Daniel suggest to King Nebuchadnezzar's steward place?

_____

_____

_____

_____

2. What happened to Daniel, Hananiah, Mishael, and Azariah after the king examined them?

_____

_____

_____

4

OVERTHROWING THE ALTAR OF FOOD ADDICTION

When you sit down to dine with a ruler, consider carefully what is [set] before you;[2] For you will put a knife to your throat, if you are a man of great appetite.

Proverbs 23:1-2

W HAT MOST OF US CALL SPIRITUAL WARFARE IS nothing short of the battle of altars. By definition and function, altars are places of exchange; they are the only legal means for spirit beings from both kingdoms to land on earth. The most important feature of an altar is the human who tends the altar. You will know an altar is involved when a person finds himself or herself in an endless cycle of repeating rituals. Without a doubt, altars are spiritual platforms for effecting spiritual encounters between humanity and divinity. Since food is spiritual, it opens the door to a person's life and world through their appetite! A person who can't let go of certain foods even when they are killing them is probably an attendant to an altar of food addiction. If you ask most Christians questions about addictions, very few of them list food in that category. The reason is simple; food is the most acceptable addiction among people of faith. Coach Scott Oatsvall calls "food addiction" in the Body of Christ "the last acceptable sin in Christendom."

FOOD ADDICTION

> Their destiny is destruction, their god is their stomach, and their glory is in their shame. Their mind is set on earthly things.
>
> —Philippians 3:19

> "Food addiction can take many forms. Symptoms include obesity, undereating, and bulimia. People often think of the term "eating disorders" when describing the disease of food addiction. Food addicts are obsessed with food, body size, and weight. We spend our days thinking about when and what we are going to eat or not eat. Binging, purging, and dieting are a way of life. The bottom line is that we can't stop thinking about eating."[1]

The above scripture from the book of Philippians ought to be scary for every believer in Jesus. According to the Apostle Paul, they are people who have made their stomachs into a god; their stomach completely runs their life. Food for them has become a powerful idol that they worship and bow to daily. To these people, Paul leaves them with a terrifying warning: their destiny is destruction, and their glory will morph into eternal shame when they finally face their maker and realize that they chose the creation (food) over the Creator, who is blessed forevermore! When your god is your stomach, there is no room for fasting to seek God's face and crucify the flesh. That will not be my portion in Jesus' name.

DOPAMINE AND FOOD ADDICTION

"If you are willing and obedient, you shall eat the best of
the land;"

—Isaiah 1:19

You don't have to be a master theologian to quickly discern the fact that the Bible makes it clear that God designed the world and built it on a healthy "cause and effect" reward system. For this reason, the Bible is full of promises from God that are lavished upon people that obey His Word. According to God's divine systems and protocol, there are promises in His Word regarding life-changing rewards waiting on people who cooperate with the laws of nature. The human body was also built on this same reward system. The chemical responsible for maintaining and fostering this eternal reward system inside the human body is a chemical known as "dopamine." Have you noticed that when you do something selfless and heroic such as rescuing a child from being hit by a car, there is a chemical rush of fulfillment that courses its way through your veins? That is the effect of dopamine.

"When acting on cravings, the brain gets a reward, a feeling of pleasure associated with the release of dopamine. The reward is what fuels our cravings and food addiction.

People with food addiction get their "fix" by eating a particular food until their brain has received all of the dopamine it was missing. The more often this cycle of craving and rewarding is repeated, the stronger it becomes and the greater the quantity of food needed each time. While four scoops of ice cream were enough three years ago, today, it may take eight scoops to experience the same level of reward. It can be almost impossible to eat in moderation when satisfying an addiction-driven craving."[2]

In my book, <u>The Battle of Altars,</u> I make it very clear that altars are places or systems of ritual. When there is repetitiveness in behavior or circumstance, a ritual is established. And wherever there is a ritual, an altar is in play. To discern what kind of altar it is, one must focus on the repetitive activity that keeps transpiring around the altar. If the ritual is an endless ritual of drugs, then the altar is an altar of addiction to drugs. In this book's context, if the ritual is an endless cycle of eating, then the altar in play is the altar of addiction to food. If you want to be honest with yourself, you may find that food is no longer just about eating to live; for many of us, eating has become about living to eat. Eating food defines everything about us. Food is, and has, become our number one idol. May God help us in Jesus' mighty name.

FOOD OFFERED TO IDOLS

But concerning the Gentiles who have believed, we wrote, having decided that they should abstain from meat sacrificed to idols and from blood and from what is strangled and from fornication."

—Acts 21:25

In the ancient world, before and after the advent of Jesus Christ, the people of that era worshiped idols by sacrificing food to them. So, in the world they lived in, sacrificing food to idols was very common. The people of the ancient world believed that eating at the altar of an idol was tantamount to becoming one with the idol. It is difficult to separate gluttony or addiction to food from demonic influence. In Jerusalem, the Apostolic Council made it clear that Gentile believers had to stay away from eating food offered to idols, drinking blood, and fornication.

Interestingly, the apostles in Jerusalem considered eating meat sacrificed to idols as grievous a sin as committing fornication. Idolizing food explains why it is so difficult for some people to let go of eating food that's not good for them. Anything you idolize has tremendous power over you. Just remember, you always become what you eat! So, if you eat junk food, don't be surprised if your health in a couple of years begins to move in the direction of the junkyard. Ask yourself this question, "Does depriving God and your family of an additional 20 years of your life not bother you at all?" It is answering this question that made me begin to move towards a deliberately designed healthy lifestyle.

LIFE APPLICATION SECTION

Memory Verse

But concerning the Gentiles who have believed, we wrote, having decided that they should abstain from meat sacrificed to idols and from blood and from what is strangled and from fornication."

—Acts 21:25

Reflections

1. Why did Gentile idol worshippers worship their idols by bringing them food?

_____

_____

_____

_____

2. Why does the misuse of Dopamine lead to terrible food addictions?

_____

_____

_____

_____

5

FINDING GOD IN WHAT YOU EAT!

And God said, "See, I have given you every herb that yields seed which is on the face of all the earth, and every tree whose fruit yields seed; to you it shall be for food.

Genesis 1:29

NOTHING IS MORE SPIRITUALLY PRICELESS THAN finding god in what you do, most especially in what you eat! Nothing influences our life more than the food we eat. If you were to roll back time to the Garden of Eden, finding God in what you ate was easy. Both man and animals had a vegetarian diet. However, God added to man's original diet to make allowances for the far-reaching implications of man's fall in the Garden of Eden. It would seem that man's body could live effortlessly on a vegetarian diet before sin and death entered. I know many Africans are going… "ouch, vegetables only!" Africans are big meat eaters but don't get me wrong; my mother would "scream murder" when I refused to eat my vegetables. However, in the beginning, it was not so! The first man and woman were gleefully vegetarian.

THE EVOLVEMENT OF MAN'S DIET!

> And God blessed Noah and his sons and said to them,
> "Be fruitful and multiply, and fill the earth. [2] The fear and
> the terror of you shall be [instinctive] in every animal of
> the land and in every bird of the air; and together with
> everything that moves on the ground, and with all the fish
> of the sea; they are given into your hand. [3] Every moving
> thing that lives shall be food for you; I give you everything,
> as I gave you the green plants and vegetables.
>
> —Genesis 9:1-3

After the global flood that God sent on earth during the days of Noah, man's diet evolved radically to include the eating of both animal and fish meat. It's clear that eating meat was not God's first plan for mankind. However, after Adam and Eve sinned and God shed blood for their atonement, it was just a matter of time before man's fallen nature would desire the flesh of something that spills blood.

Rabbi Abraham Isaac Kook, the first Chief Rabbi of Israel during the British Mandate era, offered this interpretation of Genesis 9:3:

> "Because people had sunk to an extremely low level of
> spirituality, he wrote, it was necessary that they be given
> an elevated image of themselves as compared to animals
> and that they concentrate their efforts into first improving
> relationships between people. According to Rav Kook, if
> people were denied the right to eat meat, they might eat
> the flesh of human beings due to their inability to control
> their lust for flesh. He regards the permission to slaughter
> animals for food as a "transitional tax" or temporary

dispensation until a "brighter era" is reached when people would return to vegan diets."[2]

One would think that after over 6000 years of human history, mankind would have reached this elevated image of himself in his collective consciousness. Unfortunately, Rabbi Kook did not fully understand the nature of sin; once you are infected by it, it doesn't get better without divine intervention. Mankind is still unable to control the lust of his flesh, so the "transitional tax" of eating red meat continues. Is it not interesting that there has never been a form of cancer traced to the eating of vegetables, yet red meat, has been directly connected to some types of cancers (according to the website healthline.com)? Only God knows what some animals were eating right before they became food on our plate.

Legendary Christian minister and theologian John Calvin, in his commentary on Genesis 1, suggests that men may have been permitted to eat animal meat because they were allowed to use the hides and skins of animals for clothing and shelter. He indicates, however, that he realizes that there are other opinions on this matter, and he would not take a strong position in favor of his view. His conclusion on the question of whether or not men ate meat before the Flood is that it is of "little consequence." Calvin, assuming that men ate meat before the Flood, says further in his comments on Genesis 9.3 that the reasons God explicitly granted animals for food to men were:

- To control unbridled license since the right to eat meat was granted by God after the Flood,
- Free men from having doubts about the propriety of eating meat. In other words, God validated what men had been doing without an explicit license before the Flood.

THE NEPHILIM AND CANNIBALISM

John Calvin believed that men and women were already eating animal meat long before the flood destroyed the world of men. Genesis 6 makes it clear that God was grieved by the rapid moral degradation of mankind, as the seed of men mingled with the seed of the fallen angels, producing a very violent race of giants known as the Nephilim. According to some biblical scholars, these Nephilim were carnivores with serious cannibalistic tendencies. It would seem that they taught men the depraved practice of cannibalism- where humans eat the flesh of other humans.

> There were Nephilim (men of stature, notorious men) on the earth in those days—and also afterward—when the sons of God lived with the daughters of men, and they gave birth to their children. These were the mighty men who were of old, men of renown (great reputation, fame). 5 The LORD saw that the wickedness (depravity) of man was great on the earth, and that every imagination or intent of the thoughts of his heart were only evil continually. 6The Lord regretted that He had made mankind on the earth, and He was [deeply] grieved in His heart. 7 So the LORD said, "I will destroy (annihilate) mankind whom I have created from the surface of the earth—not only man, but the animals and the crawling things and the birds of the air—because it [deeply] grieves Me [to see mankind's sin] and I regret that I have made them."
>
> —Genesis 6:4-6

The book of Enoch goes into great detail describing the abominable practices of these Nephilim (giants), including their cannibalistic tendencies. What is abundantly clear in the book of Enoch is that these Nephilim were staunch eaters of animal meat. So, it's most likely that they taught the men and women of Noah's day to eat all kinds of meat. It's also likely that "fallen" men and women were eating meat and not just sacrificing it to the LORD as Able did in Genesis 4, long before the days of Noah. However, the practice of eating all kinds of meat exploded during the reign of the Nephilim. This race of soul-less giants had an insatiable desire for meat and blood.

WHAT DID JESUS EAT?

> The Son of Man has come eating and drinking, and you say, 'Look, a man who is a glutton and a [heavy] wine-drinker, a friend of tax collectors and sinners [including non-observant Jews].'
>
> —Luke 7:33-34

What did Jesus eat? Isn't this the million-dollar question all of us want answered? Even though the first Adam was a vegetarian, the New Testament shows us that the Lord Jesus Christ ate meat, fish, and vegetables. He even ate unleavened bread and later admitted that He is the living bread of life. Additionally, Jesus also drank wine- not grape juice as some religious zealots would have you believe. If you have ever been to Israel, you would quickly realize how stupid "the grape juice" argument is. Wine is an integral part of almost every Jewish meal. It's culturally expected that if both non-observant Jews and religious observers invite you to a meal, the wine will be one of the main items. It was the same in Jesus' day. As a matter of fact, the culturally acceptable drinking of wine and eating of bread was so ingrained into ancient Jewish culture that it found its way into powerful prayers of blessing such as the "Hamotzi" and the

"HaGafen." Here is the 'Hamotzi' prayer said daily in Israel, *"Blessed are You, LORD our God, King of the universe, who brings forth bread from the earth."* Hebrew transliteration is *"Barukh ata Adonai Eloheinu, melekh ha'olam, hamotzi lehem min ha'aretz."* And then there is the 'HaGafen' prayer which is also said daily in Israel, *"Blessed are You, LORD our God, King of the universe, who creates the fruit of the vine."* Hebrew transliteration is *"Barukh ata Adonai Eloheinu, Melekh ha'olam, bo're p'ri hagefen."*

> Jesus said to them, "Come and have breakfast." None of
> the disciples dared to ask Him, "Who are You?" They knew
> [without any doubt] that it was the Lord.
>
> —John 21:12

What would you do if you woke up one morning and found Jesus in your kitchen, and he said to you, "Come and have breakfast?" I believe many of us would faint from the shock of finding Jesus in our kitchen cooking breakfast. This scripture is almost sacrilegious for some religious Christians who can't bring themselves to believe that the God and Savior of the whole world would have time for such mundane earthly tasks such as making breakfast. However, that is precisely what Jesus was doing right after He rose from the dead. You would think that He would have far more critical things to do than prepare breakfast for His wavering disciples! Oh boy, the more I come to know Him, the more I fall in love with Jesus! I wish the Bible told us what Jesus prepared for breakfast, but I can tell you this much; being both God incarnate and an observant Jewish man, the Lord Jesus' breakfast was kosher. You can forget about Jesus serving pork; it's an unclean food in Judaism.

> And when He had said this, He showed them His hands
> and His feet. While they still could not believe it because
> of their joy and amazement, He said to them, "Have you

anything here to eat?" They gave Him a piece of a broiled fish; [43] and He took it and ate it in front of them.

—Luke 24:40-43

We have already demonstrated that eating in scripture is a spiritual exercise of worship, so one of the first things Jesus Christ did after He rose from the dead was to ask for something to eat. It is a very interesting request to make for a man who had just been raised from the dead. But why did Jesus make it? I believe the Lord did it to demonstrate to His disciples and the rest of the world that He was not a spirit but a resurrected man, inside a resurrected body that could eat the food of men. However, for the sake of our study, I am more interested in what Jesus ate more than why He ate it. The Bible says that they gave him a piece of a "broiled fish."

BROILED VS. FRIED FISH?

After the resurrection, Jesus ate broiled fish. It makes you pause before you eat that deep-fried fish from the South that we all like to eat. Why would the master of the universe eat broiled fish and not the good-old-fried fish? Perhaps the article below from health.com might shed some much-needed light.

> "Eating fish has been tied with lower heart disease rates, stroke, depression, and Alzheimer's disease. But how you eat may be the real key to reaping its benefits. Recent research from the University of Pittsburgh School of Medicine concluded that study volunteers who regularly ate fish had larger brain volumes in regions associated with memory and cognition, but only if the fish is baked or broiled, not fried. Baking and broiling are also better for

your waistline. For example, a dozen fried shrimp can pack 280 calories, versus a mere 85 calories for 12 shrimp that have been steamed or broiled. To make up the difference, you would have to spend about 25 minutes on the elliptical. So, if fish and chips are your usual go-to, try lightening it up."[3]

Do you honestly believe the founders of health.com know more about the benefits of eating broiled fish versus fried fish than the God who created the fish? I don't think so! However, their analysis of the difference in "food value" between broiled fish versus fried fish just authenticates why the creator of the universe ate broiled fish after He rose from the dead. It's truly exciting to find God in what you eat!

WILD LOCUST AND HONEY

For John the Baptist has come neither eating bread nor drinking wine, and you say, 'He has a demon!'

—Luke 7:33

Now this same John had clothing made of camel's hair and a [wide] leather band around his waist; and his food was locusts and wild honey.

—Matthew 3:4

The greatest prophet of them all, John the Baptist, ate wild locust and honey. That shows us that there are various *"foods by God"* that we can eat, which will not compromise our physical health and spiritual vitality.

"The idea of eating locusts or grasshoppers is repulsive to many, but keep in mind that most think nothing of eating a cow or a chicken's flesh. It's a matter of mindset. In ancient Greece and Rome, fried locusts, cicadas, and grasshoppers were considered a delicacy superior to the best meat or fish. These insects have enormous nutritional value. Grasshoppers, for example, are 60% protein versus chicken or beef at about 20%. According to author Christopher Nyerges, "When hordes of locusts destroy acres of crops, farmers should be counting their blessings and rapidly collecting locusts. After all, the locusts are a much higher protein source than the grains they're devouring. Locusts are a good source of protein, vitamins, and minerals."[4]

Where did the prophet John the Baptist get the idea that eating wild honey and locusts was a good idea? Most importantly, how did he know that eating wild honey and locusts was very healthy and nutritious? The answer stares us in the face. John was a very observant Jew who was well-read in the Torah. He knew that God had identified locusts and wild honey as sources of healthy and divinely approved foods. Maybe he was well vested in the following passage from the book of Leviticus.

> Yet of all winged insects that walk on all fours you may eat those which have legs above their feet with which to leap on the ground. [22] Of these you may eat: the whole species of migratory locust, of bald locust, of cricket, and of grasshopper.
>
> —Leviticus 11:21-22

LIFE APPLICATION SECTION

Memory Verse

And when He had said this, He showed them His hands and His feet. While they still could not believe it because of their joy and amazement, He said to them, "Have you anything here to eat?" They gave Him a piece of a broiled fish; [43] and He took it and ate it in front of them.

—Luke 24:40-43

Reflections

1. What is the difference between broiled fish and fried fish?

_____

_____

_____

_____

2. Describe John the Baptist's diet?

_____

_____

_____

_____

"Therefore, I tell you, do not worry about your life, what you will eat or drink; or about your body, what you will wear. Is not life more than food, and the body more than clothes? ...But seek first His Kingdom and His righteousness

Math 6:29, 33 NLT

SECTION TWO

SCIENTIFIC AND MEDICAL PATHOLOGIES BEHIND FOOD ADDICTION, CELLULAR HEALTH, AND WEIGHT LOSS

Coach Scott Oatsvall

So then, whether you eat or drink or whatever you do, do all to the glory of [our great] God.

I Corinthians 10:31

6

WE ARE IN A HEALTH CRISIS

I N AMERICA, WE SPEND APPROXIMATELY 17% OF OUR
GDP on five diseases; CANCER, heart disease, high cholesterol,
diabetes, and obesity. And the fact is, 70% of all known curable
and reversible diseases are preventable. You may have heard the
saying, "An ounce of prevention is worth a pound of cure!" so let's
take a look at the numbers.

In reviewing reports from the CDC (Center for Disease Control),
you can see numbers like this as it relates to causes of death in the
U.S.:

1. Heart disease: 659,041 2. Cancer: 599,601
3. Accidents (unintentional injuries): 173,040
4. Chronic lower respiratory diseases: 156,979
5. Stroke (cerebrovascular diseases): 150,005
6. Alzheimer's disease: 121,499
7. Diabetes: 87,647
8. Nephritis, nephrotic syndrome, and nephrosis: 51,565
9. Influenza and pneumonia: 49,783
10. Intentional self-harm (suicide): 47,511

Source: Mortality in the United States, 2019, data table for figure 2 from CDC

With the emergence of the COVID-19 virus and its various strains, it is another cause of death added to the list. The data shows, those in poor health have a much higher risk for death and severe health issues related to this virus than those who are healthier with healthy immune systems.

Why is it that 70% of all known curable and reversible diseases are preventable? Because it is related to lifestyle, how a person chooses to live his or her life. For years the #1 preventable health condition was smoking. I am convinced that even smokers would admit how unhealthy smoking is, whether they have been able to quit or not. Do you know the #1 preventable health condition, pushing smoking into the #2 spot? The answer would be carrying excess body FAT! Being OVER FAT has now been in that #1 slot for several years.

The reason these diseases can be related to lifestyle is that the body is created with a specific design in how it operates best, such as:

The body is designed to carry only a certain amount of fat.

Fat gets a bad rap because the body does need a certain amount to be healthy, but it must be kept within those healthy ranges for gender, age, and body type. Having too little or having too much is a health problem. In the American culture, the focus is on being over fat since 70-80% of our adult population is considered overweight or obese. Being under fat or what we commonly call "skinny fat" comes typically in the form of eating disorders labeled as anorexic, bulimia, or a blend of those two, with cases continuing to increase. Don't kid yourself though, overeating is also an eating disorder, and any disordered way of eating creates health issues.

Our health crisis is nothing new and directly correlates to our unhealthy lifestyles and the increase of obesity in our country. The CDC and the WHO (World Health Organization) data shows that since the mid-1970s, obesity has been on a consistent and steady rise among adults and children.

The body is designed to be hydrated.

Did you know that drinking water is not an option or a suggestion for the body, but it is a critical health need? Our body's make-up, on average, is said to be two-thirds water. The make-up of our trillions and trillions of cells (no one is sure exactly how many cells a human being has) is 70% water. That means there is intracellular water and extracellular water. Understand, cells need the presence of water to function correctly.

The body is designed to move.

It seems there are too many people who view exercise, activity, or movement as something to do when I feel like losing some weight. Nothing can be further from the truth: in fact, losing weight (or should I say fat loss) is simply a side benefit. The real benefit comes from the healing properties movement brings to the body. Do you want to significantly reduce incidences of serious diseases like cancer (up to 50%) or heart disease (up to 30%)? Then get moving since moderate activity for as little as thirty minutes a day, five to six days a week, directly correlates to reducing the occurrence of these diseases. Movement is not a problem (e.g., I hate exercise); it is a blessing. In reality, all of us appreciate the ability to move. The real problem is when a person's movement becomes limited, or even worse; a person becomes immobile. I can't imagine anyone ever choosing to live that way. Each of us should take advantage of our ability to move and learn to appreciate movement if we do not already.

Exercise and movement also come in basic strength exercises that will help with muscle and bone health. Bones are your framework, and muscles do the work of the body. It is not about simply lifting weights and bulking up (which is not the LT360 way). It is about maintaining health and wellness through lean muscle mass. I have heard that a person who does not engage in some form of basic muscular strength exercises will lose 1% muscle mass each year, beginning in those middle-age years. We usually think of the middle-age years beginning in our mid 40's. Can you imagine losing 1% each year for the remaining years of a person's life? That could end up being many years and create a myriad of health issues.

The body is designed to use energy.

This energy comes in the form of the calories we take in through either the foods we eat or the beverages we drink. Why has the obesity rate among our children and adults increased steadily over decades now? Because too many people have created an energy imbalance.

Think of it this way. Our bodies need energy, and our bodies are also designed for survival. The body is designed to only use so much energy/calories each day based on our BMR - Basal Metabolic Rate (more on this later). If we take in more than we can use, our bodies won't "waste" it but will store it. In this sense, the body responds like, "you gave it to me, so at some point, I will need it in the future." The body stores it as fat, which we think of negatively, but the body views it as "future food." The problem in our culture is people rarely find themselves needing stored fat as future food. Not too many of us will be on that deserted island and need stored food to sustain us until rescued. What is needed is to bring the imbalance back into a balanced state.

If we are not working with our body's design, we significantly increase our chance of disease and sickness. Of course, nobody wants to be sick and end up a statistic! None of us want to be a burden on our family, lose our independence, and suffer from a chronic illness or disease that we can prevent. BAD HEALTH IS NEVER INTENTIONAL!

Why does our health continue to be put on the back burners of our lives until we have a health crisis? Here are a few key reasons; how many sound familiar?

1. Time
    Time is an excuse for neglect. People in a hurry don't have time to care for themselves or improve their health. Most people are sprinting just to stand still!

2. Excuses
    Every day is an excuse for bad habits. You look around one day and wonder how things got this way.

3. Problems
    Problems seem to give purpose to your existence. In the process of focusing on problems, environments go dark, and people grow discouraged.

4. Fear
    Fear is the most paralyzing emotion most people face. Fear will keep you parked in the middle of the road.

5. Lack of knowledge
    Most people have very little understanding of nutrition and how the body heals and repairs itself.

So, as you read this book, here are five questions to ask as you evaluate your health:

1. What am I willing to do to make my health improve?
2. Do my life and health truly matter?
3. At what time in my life did I feel my best?
4. What things seem to take too much time? How might I remedy that?
5. What five behaviors might make my health better?

Before you can get healthy at the cellular level, we all must stop and take an honest assessment of where we are and where we want to go; mentally, physically, and spiritually. The question is, what can you do to keep your immune system strong and avoid the next medical crisis that might lead to you becoming one of the statistics. And, if you are currently fighting something – change things now. "You don't have to be healthy to get started, but you do have to get started to be healthy!" A strong immune system will not only keep you healthier but will also help your body heal. Remember, "It's hard to make a healthy cell sick!" You do this by getting healthy at the cellular level.

SO LET'S GET STARTED…

LIFE APPLICATION SECTION

Memory Verse

Beloved, I pray that in every way you may succeed and prosper and be in good health [physically], just as [I know] your soul prospers [spiritually].

—3 John 2:2

Reflections

1. According to the CDC, what is the leading cause of death in America?

_____

_____

_____

_____

2. What are you willing to do to improve your health improve?

_____

_____

_____

_____

7

WHY WE GET SICK AS WE AGE

I THINK IT WAS GEORGE BURNS WHO SAID, "IF I KNEW I was going to live this long, I would have taken better care of my body!" Ever wonder why older people often contract diseases? It all comes down to how healthy or unhealthy our body's cells are, which is related to how healthy or unhealthy they are regenerating or reproducing. Before we talk about cellular health, let's look at the current state of elderly health. Roughly half of all people today die from cardiovascular disease. Another third or more die from some form of cancer. But I believe these are not age-related diseases. As I said previously, they are diet and lifestyle-related. Without changes in diet, medical costs will continue to soar; older Americans will continue to get sick and not enjoy their golden years.

We have come to accept this current accelerated aging process as the new normal. We accept putting on weight each year, known as "creeping weight," because we are getting older. We accept the aches and pains and loss of overall well-being because it is what we now think is "supposed to happen." Of course, as we age, we will have more significant limitations than what we had in our earlier years. Still, it can happen in a much more natural way than in this accelerated manner that is currently happening in our culture. As we get older, do you honestly think we must "accept" the loss of feeling good or have less energy? Of course not, and it can be put back under your control.

One of the most rewarding parts of my job is witnessing my older clients' transformation after they decide to take charge of their health and embrace the structure of the LT360 lifestyle. As anyone can see from all of our testimonies, many seniors have overcome significant health challenges and are now experiencing something they never thought possible; a whole new level of health and wellness as well as more personal independence. They have not only added years to their life but have enriched their quality of life. They feel better, and they can do more. You can not put a price on how you feel!

How and Why Does LT360 Structure Work?

As I said earlier, it all comes down to the cells in our body. When our cells are sick, we get sick. When our cells are healthy, we are healthy. Science tells us that free radicals can damage vital cellular components, including the body's DNA or cell membranes. Cells may then function poorly or die. However, when our cells operate the way God designed them, we enjoy optimal health and a slow, healthy aging process. So know that you are about to find a structure to change your health and your future forever.

What we call fat, our body calls "future food."

Your responsibility is to create an environment where your cells will regenerate in a healthy manner which happens when you work with your body's design through a healthy lifestyle. When you live in an unhealthy manner, cells will not be as healthy and will regenerate as unhealthy. Look under a microscope, and you can see the difference between a healthy cell and an unhealthy cell. A healthy cell is more round with its membrane intact. An unhealthy cell has a distorted membrane, one we would label as a "flat" cell.

Have you ever wondered why your grandparents seemed to be healthier than our generation? Probably not. One of the reasons is their lifestyles were probably more active than ours. The air they breathed was cleaner, the food they ate was cleaner without the added hormones, pesticides, synthetics, and depleted soils of foods today.

Your grandparents probably got between seven to eight hours of sleep each night. And although the stress and anxiety they experienced were different from ours, they didn't have to deal with a world filled with social media, the internet, cell phones, and 24-hou negative news cycles. And in all reality, life was much simpler.

We live in a world today where stress and working 50, 60, and 70 hours a week is normal. And not only is working like this praised, in many cases, it's also expected. Add to this, stressors from such areas as home and family life, finances, and relationships begin to take their toll. As research and technology continue to advance, scientists are discovering many health problems caused by stress exhaustion and its effects on the body.

There are two types of stress; one positive and one negative. Positive or good stress is referred to as eustress. Negative stress is called distress. Eustress is when a person gets excited or sometimes referred to as the "pre-game jitters" or "butterflies." The body has the same physical response associated with any stress, but eustress is related to a positive experience and can help a person perform better. Distress, on the other hand, requires good coping tools.

The body has a natural, built-in alarm system to deal with life's stressors. The design is based on a short-term attack from "predators or aggressors," commonly referred to as the "flight or fight" response. There are automatic physical responses such as increased heart rate, increased breathing, increased adrenaline, and cortisol release, which are all intended to increase focus, alertness, and the body's ability to respond to the attack. Once the danger passes, the body returns to normal.

In this day and age, these "attacks" come in all shapes and forms. Unfortunately, these are not so much short-term as they have become long, drawn-out sieges from various pressure points related to our lives and work. Dealing with difficult life or family situations, work-related issues, and the busy schedule demands life places on each of us can hinder our body's ability to move from a highly stressed state back to a normal state.

🍎

Positive or good stress is referred to as eustress.
Negative stress is called distress.

Part of a long-term stressed state involves increased cortisol levels, which increase blood sugar levels, leading to weight gain and higher levels of belly fat. Cortisol and fat burning do not go hand in hand and can hinder your weight loss goals. How does this work?

1. Cortisol is catabolic, meaning it causes the breakdown of muscle tissue. Muscle is too expensive to lose.
2. Elevated stress levels can lead to out-of-control food cravings and the feeling of always being hungry. That is never fun.
3. Stress also inhibits your body's ability to release stored fat as food or fuel. When you are under constant stress, neurologically and biologically speaking, it is similar to smoking cigarettes or drinking alcohol every day. And we all know how that will likely end up.

Of course, stress can affect your sleep cycle as well. Lack of sleep can also increase cortisol levels, and thus a vicious cycle begins. I am stressed, I can't turn off my mind, and I don't sleep.

I don't sleep, and that increases my stress. Never for one moment think you are wasting time when sleeping. It is during sleep that the body heals and repairs itself.

What happens when you become sleep-deprived? How many of these symptoms do you manifest?

1) Fatigue, lethargy, and lack of motivation
2) Moodiness and irritability
3) Reduced creativity and problem-solving skills
4) Less ability or even inability to cope with stress
5) Reduced immunity, more frequent colds, and infections
6) Concentration and memory problems
7) Weight gain related to grehlin (hunger hormone) and leptin (energy balance hormone)
8) Impaired motor skills and the increased chance of accidents
9) Difficulty in making decisions
10) Increased risk of diabetes, heart disease, and other health problems

What happens during those seven-nine hours of sleep?

1) Tissue growth and repair
2) Energy is restored, providing energy to the brain and body
3) Hormones are released, which are essential for growth, development (including muscle development), and appetite control (sleep-deprived = weight gain)
4) Supports daytime performance and focus
5) Contributes to a healthy immune system

As you can see, getting the proper amount of sleep is what allows you to enjoy life during your waking hours (one study recommended 7 1/2 hours for adults as ideal, though some may still need more).

Remember, you are not alone. Stress gets the best of all of us from time to time. Responding to the immediate physical effects of stress can help lessen stress's long-term and mental effects. But if you don't learn to get your stress under control, it's nearly impossible to be healthy, happy, and whole, and it will be almost impossible to lose that stubborn fat. Since there is no such thing as a totally stress-free life, the key is learning how to handle life's stressors positively, which comes from having a healthy lifestyle.

The constant bombardment of stressors is why it is very challenging to stay healthy in the world we live in today. It is why it is so important to make your health your priority from the moment you wake up to the time you go to bed. When people are rushed, there is no time to create a calm mind and a physically active body, so many people report high anxiety and stress levels. The medical term for this is called "stress exhaustion."

If you don't schedule time for your health, it won't happen. If you don't plan to keep yourself healthy, then you are, by default, planning to get sick. If you are tired of properly fueling your body every day, then just imagine what it would look like if you forgot to fill up your car with gas when it is on empty. It would stop working! If you honestly believe that you can get away with neglecting your health, the only one you have fooled is you! You undoubtedly didn't fool your body! And it won't be long before you see the red flags that will soon turn into chronic illness and disease.

If you think it is a lot of work to stay healthy, you will be shocked at how much work it is to regain your health. And I know first-hand it is a great deal more work trying to be healthy, happy, and whole while you are sick. That is no way to live. This isn't a practice life! This is your only chance at life. You must make every effort to get all that you can from it. And if you will commit to your health, you will be able to maintain your balance, flexibility, independence, and mind. These are gifts that can quickly be taken from you if you don't strive to keep them. You will have more time with family and loved ones enjoying each other and creating memories that will last longer than the pain of discipline it took to stay healthy. Remember, the pain of regret can last forever!

LIFE APPLICATION SECTION

Memory Verse

> Now when Isaac was old and his eyes were too dim to see, he called his elder [and favorite] son Esau and said to him, "My son." And Esau answered him, "Here I am." ² Isaac said, "See here, I am old; I do not know when I may die.
>
> —Genesis 27:1-2

Reflections

1. What do we mean when we say Cortisol is catabolic?

_____

_____

_____

_____

2. Why do most people get sicker the older they get?

_____

_____

_____

_____

Then God said, "Look! I have given you every seed- bearing plant throughout the earth and all the fruit trees for your food.

Genesis 1:29

8

GRACEFUL AGING

WHEN YOU LOOK AT YOURSELF IN THE MIRROR, does your reflection make you feel older? Maybe you've put on weight, and you can't fit into your jeans anymore, do you think, "WOW! I look great!?"

Is your body holding you back from playing with your kids, grandkids, your dog, taking walks, or just sitting comfortably? Getting older is something that most of us don't look forward to, but why? Because it's painful, things fall apart. Joints ache. We start to get wrinkles. We move slower. Believe me; it doesn't have to be this way. There is one BIG secret to aging gracefully...I know I'm beginning to sound like a broken record, but it's called Cellular Health. Let that term sink deep down in your spirit.

Remember the Bible story of building your house on sand and building your house on the rock? When you build your house on sand, and the rain picks up, the streams rise, and the winds blow, it washes away. If you build your house on the rock, it will stand strong against the storm because of its firm foundation. Your body works the same way. If you are using building blocks such as veggies, proteins, drinking lots of water, exercising, and top-quality supplements, you are building your body "on the rock." It's not just building but also eliminating toxic and inflammatory foods as well. Your body will be able to stand against sickness, disease, and injury because cellular health creates strong cells. Strong cells are healthy cells, and healthy cells age SLOWLY, making you look and feel younger.

So, as you can see, having a structure and framework to get healthy is vital. But what if you have a family history of health challenges like I did? Is it possible to use this framework to change your family's health? I SAY YES!!! Let me illustrate this point.

Do you remember the days when you had to rush home from school or work so you could be at the dinner table to eat the evening meal with your family? The evening meal time was a sacred event for many of us! There was no excuse to miss dinner. The phone wasn't to be answered, and the TV was off while people were eating. My wife and I both came from not very well-to-do families, so our evening meals weren't considered "King's food" by any stretch of the imagination. In fact, my Sunday dinner often consisted of lots of casseroles, and I remember fried potatoes and wish meat sandwiches (two pieces of bread and WISH you had some meat!). But what I remember more than the food was the consistency of the experience. I remember the gentle way my grandmother taught us table manners, the conversations, and the love that developed between children and parents (and, in my case, grandparents). It seems hard to find today. Sadly, America ranks 33rd out of 35 nations when it comes to eating family meals together consistently.

So, what is the big deal about eating family meals together? Take a look at what you and your family will benefit from if you eat at least four meals every week together. The Benefits of the Family Table - American College of Pediatrics studies show that your child may be:

- 35% less likely to experience eating disorders
- 24% more likely to eat healthier foods
- 12% less likely to be overweight

It is also known that they experience:

- Fewer episodes of depression (improved psychological well- being)
- Less delinquency, alcohol, drug, and tobacco abuse
- Greater academic achievement
- Delayed sexual activity
- More instances where they can say their parents are proud of them

There is a greater likelihood of boosting their vocabulary through dinner conversation than by reading. Interestingly, researchers like Howard LeWine, M.D. Chief Medical Editor, Harvard Health Publishing, have found that meals eaten in front of the TV or with people on their cell phones do not carry the same mental health benefits as those eaten "unplugged." One survey found that the 9-14-year olds who ate dinner with their families most frequently are more fruits and vegetables and less soda and fried foods. Their diets also had higher amounts o many vital nutrients like calcium, iron, and fiber.

A family meal is a perfect time to introduce a child to new foods and different tastes (we know, we have six kids). Gwen and I have been amazed at what our kids will eat when we started eating healthier.

Try eating "unplugged," enjoy your food and the company!

What are the benefits of family mealtime which have been demonstrated for children of all ages? Better grades, healthier eating habits, closer relationships to parents and siblings, ability to resist negative peer pressure, resilience in the face of life's problems, to name a few. All these are outcomes of simply sharing dinner regularly.

What else can families do that takes only about an hour a day and packs such a punch?

How to age gracefully:

1. **Have a plan to get healthy.**
   A plan for healthy living can help you make healthy behaviors part of your life. Start by keeping it simple. Expand your strategies as you can over time. There can also be comfort in knowing you are doing what you can to reduce your risk for disease and other health problems. Include any new goals you have set for yourself.

2. **Be committed to your health.**
   Getting healthy is all about commitment. There is no way around it. Being interested and being committed are two very different things. I know it takes courage, but there is no shortcut when it comes to your health. Your health is the greatest gift you have! YOUR HEALTH IS YOUR WEALTH!

3. **Trust the process.**
   There is no such thing as perfection when it comes to health: it's always a work in progress. Your health is dynamic, constantly changing, as we, too, as individuals, constantly change and shift. Mistakes happen. You are going to do things that you later regret. It can be very painful at times. Successful people have learned how to accept these difficult moments and turn them into springboards that take their health to the next level. They use the proven process to keep motivated and inspired to keep going! Trust the process, don't rush it.

4. **Stay connected to a community of like-minded people.**

   The most important thing to remember is to stay close with the ones walking the trail with you. For the LT360 community, it is reading their email lessons, connecting with the group on Facebook, and coming in for coaching evaluations that are so important.

5. **Keep curiosity alive.**

   Successful people never get tired of discovering new information and being educated. They make an effort to see every morning as a new opportunity to grow. Like treasure hunters, they look for and appreciate the beauty that dwells in the things they learn.

   Overall, healthy people know that their health rests on commitment and that commitment is about consistency—the consistency of being open and honest to follow the plan. This requires another skill and attitude that is fundamental to experience lasting health—self-acceptance. We cannot accept others or even forgive others if we don't first accept and forgive ourselves. We cannot achieve cellular health if we are not taking full responsibility for our actions, decisions, and words.

LIFE APPLICATION SECTION

Memory Verse

> Although Moses was a hundred and twenty years old when
> he died, his eyesight was not dim, nor his natural strength
> abated.
>
> —Deuteronomy 34:7

Reflections

1. What do you see when you look at yourself in the mirror?

_____

_____

_____

_____

2. Why is your health your wealth?

_____

_____

_____

_____

Beloved, I pray that you may prosper in all things and be in health, just as your soul prospers.

III John 1:2

9

CAN WE REALLY LIVE DISEASE-FREE?

AGING GRACEFULLY IS ONE THING, BUT WHAT about lowering your risk for disease and sickness? The sad reality is, people are getting sicker despite the advancements in research and medical treatments. We all know someone who has been affected by illness and disease. It can be scary to have a close family member or friend receive a diagnosis such as diabetes or cancer.

Even though there are many diseases, it doesn't mean that you don't have any control over your risk. We have found that lifestyle factors play a role in the risk of almost all diseases, and you can make changes in your daily habits to reduce your risk. These lifestyle changes might seem trivial initially, but healthy habits can add up over time to protect your overall health and wellness. So, what are those lifestyle changes going to affect when you start your journey of health?

Developing a robust immune system is the place to start. Immune strength comes from the way that you are treating your body, beginning with hydration. To understand the importance of being hydrated and cellular health, let's cover some "Cell Basics." Cells are:

1. The basic building blocks of all living things
2. The smallest structural and functional unit of an organism
3. Numbered in the trillions within the human body.
4. Constantly dividing, dying, and regenerating

A dehydrated cell's membrane becomes less porous, which will lead to an increase of toxins and acids. It also hampers the flow of nutrients and hormones into the cells and waste flowing out. When waste products such as oxidants cannot leave the cell, damage occurs to the cell.

*You **can** control your risk for disease!*

On average, our bodies are said to be two-thirds water. Cells themselves are 70% water. Here's how the body uses water:

1. The digestive system must have water to break down and digest food (vitamins and nutrients).
2. Proper digestion detoxifies the liver and kidneys and carries waste away
3. Red blood cells use water in collecting oxygen in the lungs
4. Regulates the body's temperature by controlling the body's thermostat
5. Regulates blood pressure
6. Serves as a bonding adhesive to the structure of a cell
7. Generates energy as it flows through the cell's membrane
8. Necessary for the metabolic breakdown of ATP, another source of cellular energy
9. Drinking at least 8-10 eight-ounce glasses of water per day could significantly reduce joint and back pain for 80% of sufferers

10. Drinking at least five eight-ounce glasses of water can reduce the risk of colon cancer, breast cancer, and bladder cancer

To also understand the importance of hydration, one must realize the problems associated with being dehydrated. Most Americans are walking around dehydrated and do not even know it. One study concluded that 75% of Americans are dehydrated. In our senior population over the age of 65, dehydration was one of the most frequent causes of hospitalization.

Dehydration begins with not drinking enough water, but it is not the only factor since plenty of big water drinkers can be dehydrated. Everything works together in how you live to make sure the body can uptake the water and not simply pass through you.

Dehydration is also prevalent among those who drink caffeinated sodas, coffees, teas, and alcohol. These beverages have diuretic properties which means they are pushing water out of the body. When people drink these types of beverages, the toxins in these drinks need high amounts of water to be adequately filtered and flushed from the body. These drinks can also increase acid levels, which puts more stress on the kidneys. They also increase the rate of urine production, which means the water in these drinks is eliminated before the cells can use it.

When you realize that, on average, Americans are getting 21% of their daily caloric intake from beverages such as these, it is easier to understand why it is a problem. Since water is a need (not an option or a suggestion), and these beverages are certainly not a need, you realize the importance of prioritizing water as your "beverage of choice." Be reminded that more often than not, feeling a little weak, having a headache, being hungry is the body telling you it needs water, not food.

Problems associated with even slight dehydration include:

- Lack of energy, feelings of lethargy
- Short-term memory loss
- Trouble with basic math
- Difficulty focusing on a computer screen or a printed page
- Slows down metabolism

Dehydration is associated with increasing histamine, inhibiting insulin, joint pain, headaches, weight gain, fatigue, high blood pressure, increasing blood sugars, ulcers, food cravings, irritability, depression, anxiety, and kidney disease. These are the reasons why we start with hydration.

You can live without food longer than you can live without water!

Another crucial area is to ensure that you are eating all of the nutrients (vitamins and minerals) that will support your overall health. Increase your consumption of fruits and vegetables, eat healthy sources of fats and lean meats, and stick with whole grains and sprouted grains instead of refined sugar and white flour. For example, minerals help transport water into the cells, where they activate enzymes. Enzymes are the basis of all biological processes in the body, from digestion to hormone secretion to cognition. Are you beginning to see within the design of our bodies that everything works together and is connected? What God has created is truly amazing.

Physical activity level is also essential. So make sure you are moving your body around each day. The great news is you don't have to kill yourself and hate the process. Basic body movement such as walking can do wonders for you. Start with where you are and build from there.

You can use other supports to strengthen your immune system, including certain supplements like Vitamin C and MSM found in the Heal & Recovery Powder. As you are changing your lifestyle, you can use the recipes we have created on social media on our Facebook page (search for LT360 or Coach Scott Oatsvall). These recipes will make it easier for you to boost your immune system through healthy food choices.

Another change to consider is to eliminate as many toxic and inflammatory foods as possible: food such as refined grains and refined sugars. Some people that suffer from autoimmune disorders may need to eliminate dairy and glute altogether.

When toxins increase, it is much harder for the body to fight illness and disease. As a result, a disease might develop because of toxin exposure. Eliminate these foods whenever possible to support your cellular health.

*Our bodies were made to **move**!*

Reduce and manage stress levels.

High levels of stress have been linked with the development of many diseases. By decreasing stress levels, you can reduce your risk for disease and sickness at the same time. The first step is to identify those stressors and see which ones can be controlled or removed or cannot be controlled. It would be best if you talked with key people; for example, a work supervisor might help alleviate specific work-related stressors.

Aside from following LT360's **5 to Thrive** cellular health program described in this book, other suggestions to deal with life's stressors in a positive way include some of these strategies:

Short term:

1. Escape/take a break/go outside
2. Quick activity/walk break
3. Breathing exercises
4. Stretch/relax muscles
5. Splash cool water on the face
6. Warm-up/rub hands together and place over eyes
7. Gently massage face and ears
8. Laugh/think of something amusing

Long term:

1. Adopt a hobby
2. Eliminate or reduce caffeine
3. Utilize aromatherapy
4. Learn relaxation techniques
5. Don't overuse or abuse alcohol or drugs
6. Don't overextend yourself; learn to say "No."
7. I also make daily prayer and scripture reading part of my life; this has helped me to feel less stressed.

By combining these basic strategies, you will be able to support your overall health and reduce the risk of certain lifestyle diseases.

LIFE APPLICATION SECTION

Memory Verse

He also brought them out with silver and gold, and there
was none feeble among His tribes.

—Psalm 105:37

Reflections

1. Is it possible to live sick-free? Why?

_____

_____

_____

_____

2. What is the importance of being hydrated?

_____

_____

_____

_____

10

LITTLE WHITE LIES

I HAD THE PLEASURE OF ATTENDING A NUTRITION seminar years ago with some good presentations. Still, I had to laugh when one speaker—a clinical nutritionist at that—stated that one rule she requires EVERY client to follow is the "no white foods" rule.

NONE!

Really?

Of course, I understand that the rule is a good one when applied to processed "white" foods like bread, pasta, crackers, and refined sugars. However, believe it or not, this nutritionist specifically outlawed other white foods such as bananas and potatoes just because of their color! WOW!

Many WHITE foods fuel your metabolism and help you burn fat: Veggies such as onions, cauliflower, garlic, turnips, parsnips, and mushrooms are all loaded with vitamins, minerals, and fiber while containing almost zero calories. Fill your plate with these white gems, and watch your health platform rise! Other examples are white beans which are high in protein, very low glycemic (so they're easy on your blood sugar), and high fiber. As you can see, all white foods are not the devil; just know which ones are!

Let's take dairy products such as milk, cottage cheese, and other cheeses, which are all very high in protein, while other dairy products such as yogurt and kefir offer probiotics to boot! I realize that some people are sensitive to dairy, but there are still good nutritional benefits for those who are not. Then, seeds like pumpkin seeds and even white chia seeds pack a super food punch as they are rich in omega-3s, protein, antioxidants, and fiber. And lastly (but certainly not least!) are the many varieties of white fish

— another great metabolism-boosting source of protein. But here's something you may not know: while we've been told that fish is one of the healthiest food choices around (and for the most part, it is), you want to avoid farm-raised fish as much as possible.

God-made or man-made, which do you think is better?

Let's go a little deeper on my No. 1 and No. 2 public enemies: refined grains and refined sugar. I have talked about sugar's effects like a broken record, but now a recent report states that scientists have concluded that sugar is addictive. Some researchers even liken sugar to drugs or alcohol. The evidence is overwhelming and explains why some people struggle to resist or limit their refined sugar intake. (I struggled with this for years.) And yes, I was addicted!

Dr. Nicole Avena, a neuroscientist and research psychologist at Columbia University who has done a lot of work in the area of food addiction, has researched the neurotransmitters and brain receptors involved in eating. In her experiments, she has shown how overeating foods (like sugar) can produce changes in the brain and behavior that resemble addiction, like drugs and alcohol. WOW! I guess the sugar did make me do it! It's easy for some of us to steer clear of drugs, whiskey, wine, and beer. But sugar?

When you consider that there are approximately 600,000 food items in America, and 80% contain added sugar, avoiding sugar is a lot more challenging. Here is the point: If you have experienced out-of-control sugar cravings and give in from time to time, do it rarely and cautiously. Otherwise, there's a pretty good chance that your brain is going to start demanding sugar all the time! That's a voice I do not want back in my head! Keep doing your best to eat smart and avoid refined sugars as much as possible. Use honey and stevia for your sweeteners. More on that later.

Now before you throw me out with the bathwater, let's talk about the different types of sugar. Here is a good reference by nutritionist Jake Carney for the different types of sugar:

1. **Refined white sugar.** It's public enemy number one! Refined white sugar is completely stripped of all nutritional value and provides only empty calories. Furthermore, more than 65 percent of the white sugar available commercially is made from genetically modified (GMO) sugar beets. Stay away as much as possible.

2. **Brown sugar:** Commercial brown sugar is nothing more than refined white sugar with some molasses added back in for color and flavor. Don't be fooled by the color or claims. It's just as bad.

3. **Evaporated cane juice:** Made from sugar cane (as opposed to sugar beets), evaporated cane juice is slightly less refined than white sugar, and therefore retains more color, flavor, and nutrients from the sugar cane. But the only difference between commercial evaporated cane juice and white sugar is that the former goes through one less step of refinement.

4. **Cane sugar:** This sugar type is less processed than refined white sugar and still contains some of the original nutrients present in cane juice. These include amino acids, minerals, vitamins, and even some antioxidants. You also won't be exposed to the pesticides present in commercially grown sugar because it's organic. So, while a better choice than refined white sugar, remember that it's still SUGAR and should be consumed in minimal amounts.

5. **Coconut sugar:** Coconut sugar is harvested from the sap of the coconut plant through a very natural process of extracting the juice and then allowing the water to evaporate. Process-wise, it is one of the most sustainable sugar production methods, and the product also contains a small amount of fiber and other nutrients. Coconut also contains a lower percentage of fructose than the other sugars listed, making it slightly healthier than the other options.

   Other than the different types of sugars discussed above, there is one "sugar" that, in its raw form, contains a highly concentrated dose of vitamins, minerals, and other nutrients that help nourish, heal and repair your body - Honey!

6. **Honey** is the only pre-digested food on the planet and contains a concentrated dose of vitamins, minerals, and nutrients that nourish and revitalize your body. It also possesses unique antimicrobial properties that help you fight off infections. It's liquid GOLD!

   Throughout history, honey has been used to treat:

o   Coughs   o   Indigestion   o   Flu
o   Wounds   o   Fatigue   o   Burns
o   Skin infections,
    and more!

Don't be fooled by the hype of other sugars. Honey is your go-to sweetener! Stevia and Monk Fruit are also good choices for natural sweeteners.

Our bodies are designed to process "natural" food, "refined" foods, not so much!

One of the very few foods I recommended that you eliminate from your diet besides refined sugar is refined grains (white flour). However, that doesn't mean you have to eliminate all bread, baked goods, and pasta for good. For example, 100% Whole Wheat flour is an excellent alternative to white flour, but why is it better for you?
Let's look at 100% whole wheat, it…

1.   Contains more nutrients.
2.   Doesn't have bleach
3.   Has a lower impact on blood sugar
4.   Doesn't affect your metabolism and digestion the same
5.   Has higher fiber content

Both white and whole wheat flour are milled from soft wheat, red wheat, white spring wheat, or another kind of wheat. The primary difference between white and wheat flour is that white flour is heavily processed and refined. That's why it's called "refined wheat." On the other hand, 100% wheat flour retains its wholeness and is processed very little. So if you are a bread person, then the nutritional benefits of 100% whole wheat will serve you well as long as you don't have any gluten issues. The higher fiber content alone is worth making the switch. Fiber can reduce your risk of heart attack or stroke; most Americans aren't getting nearly enough fiber. Another thing worth noting is eating white flour products can lead to nutritional deficiency, which can cause chronic disease and illnesses. I'm not saying an occasional white flour product will kill you, but be mindful you have many better options. Finally, preservatives, bleach, and additives in refined white flour are added to improve the look, texture, and shelf-life and can trigger increased toxin levels in your body. So go whole wheat or sprouted wheat whenever possible.

LIFE APPLICATION SECTION

Memory Verse

You are of your father the devil, and the desires of your father you want to do. He was a murderer from the beginning, and does not stand in the truth, because there is no truth in him. When he speaks a lie, he speaks from his own resources, for he is a liar and the father of it.

—John 8:44

Reflections

1. Write down three examples of good white foods?

    _____

    _____

    _____

    _____

2. Eating foods high in fiber can reduce your risk of what disease?

    _____

    _____

    _____

11

BIG FAT LIES

W E'VE ALL HEARD THEM; THE DOES AND DON'TS of good health. Sadly, they seem to change as often as the weather. Often, the nutrition instruction given is s not incorrect, but it is usually incomplete. One of the characteristics of a lie that makes it believable is that there is some truth in it. Let's look at some of the more common and correct them with scientific facts regarding how the body is designed to function.

LIE NUMBER 1: ALL FAT IS BAD.
LET'S TAKE A CLOSER LOOK.

The central part of the fat in our diets and our bodies is in the form of triglycerides. The rest is cholesterol, waxes, and phospholipids. All triglycerides are made up of a fork-like structure called glycerol and three building blocks called fatty acids. Fatty acids are classified according to the number of double bonds they possess. Saturated fats contain no double bond, monounsaturated fats (MUFA) contain one, and polyunsaturated fats contain two or more. These fatty acids are responsible for the physical properties of the fat. As a general rule, saturated fats are solid at room temperature and tend to be derived from animal sources. One exception would be coconut oil which is a healthy fat that is solid at room temperature. Most unsaturated fats are liquid at room temperature and are usually vegetable fats like oils.

The body can make all the fatty acids it needs except for two known essential fatty acids: alpha-linolenic acid and linoleic acid. These polyunsaturated fatty acids must be supplied in the diet. Good sources of these fatty acids are vegetables and also fish.

According to a study that appeared in *Diabetes Care*, a journal published by the American Diabetes Association, a diet rich in monounsaturated fats (MUFA) may help reduce abdominal fat better than a carbohydrate-rich diet. When test subjects ate a carbohydrate-enriched diet, they tended to accumulate fat in the abdomen. When they ate a diet that had more MUFA, the abdominal fat concentration decreased, even without exercise.

Here are some MUFA rich foods?

- Olives and olive oil
- Nuts and nut oils
- Seeds and seed oils
- Grape seed oil
- Avocados

That is an excellent place to start with getting healthy fats into your diet.

Repeat after me, "IN with the good at, OUT with the BAD!"

LIE NUMBER 2: CHOLESTEROL IS BAD. LET'S TAKE A CLOSER LOOK.

Contrary to what we've been told, cholesterol is not the doorway to heart disease. It's not here to destroy our hearts! Cholesterol has many benefits to the body, including insulating neurons, building and maintaining cellular membranes, immune response, metabolizing fat-soluble vitamins, synthesizing vitamin D, producing bile, and working with the body's synthesis of many hormones. Without cholesterol, we would be dead!

Since up to 90% of cholesterol is produced from the liver, let's first talk about the liver and understand its importance to our health.

The liver is the body's largest internal organ and a true warrior for health. It is responsible for more than 500 metabolic processes, including detoxifying and purifying the blood, converting nutrients into energy, aiding in digestion, manufacturing proteins and fats, storing essential vitamins and minerals, and even helping with weight loss. Unfortunately, the data shows:

1. Over 70% of Americans are overweight and have a plethora of health problems. Being overweight has a direct connection to the health of the liver. [5]
2. It is estimated that 80 to 100 million Americans have NAFLD (Non-Alcoholic Fatty Liver Disease).[6]
3. One in 10 children in the United States is estimated to have a fatty liver. That is seven million children![7]

Let's address the fatty liver first:

A fatty liver is placed in a bear hug, smothering inside the body, forced to suffer, strain, and eventually slows down from sheer exhaustion. An overworked liver can lead to many unpleasant symptoms such as struggling to recall familiar names or words, catching every virus that goes around the office or church, and becoming exhausted by mid-afternoon. Impaired brain function ("brain fog"), a weakened immune system, and fatigue are all common symptoms of a sluggish liver.

WHAT ABOUT NON-ALCOHOLIC FATTY LIVER DISEASE (NAFLD)?

NAFLD often develops in people who are overweight or obese or have diabetes, high cholesterol, or high triglycerides. Sedentary behavior is another major contributing factor to the onset of NAFLD. NAFLD starts with no symptoms, but it will lead to NASH (Non-alcoholic Steatohepatitis) if left untreated. NASH occurs when the liver inflames; then cirrhosis can set in, leading to a myriad of problems, including a build-up of toxins in the brain.

The liver, health, and weight are all interrelated. If we overeat and become obese, then we damage the liver. If we damage the liver, then we damage our metabolism and increase the likelihood of remaining obese. Obesity leads to other health problems, which multiplies the damage to the liver and causes increased fat storage. It is a vicious circle!

If any of the fatty liver or NAFLD symptoms sound familiar, here's some good news: the liver is the only internal organ that can regenerate itself. That means, even if you're feeling worn out and run down because your liver is "sick," you do not have to stay that way. You can turn the tables on liver health. It will not happen overnight, but it can happen in as little as 8-12 weeks of being consistent in doing the right things, LT360 style!

The health of your liver is critical to your overall well-being!

Now back to the liver and its real relationship with cholesterol.

The liver is careful to ensure the body always has enough, producing 1000-1400 milligrams each day. That is why it's essential to understand that most of the time, cholesterol is a liver issue, NOT a dietary problem. Dietary cholesterol is a relative drop in the bucket.

And besides, the liver has sensitive feedback mechanisms that regulate cholesterol production in response to how much you get from your diet. Eat more cholesterol, make less in the liver. Eat less cholesterol, make more in the liver.

Now, if cholesterol is so important, why do we worry about it at all? How has it garnered such a bad reputation for giving us heart attacks?

It's called the "Statin Drug" industry. Enough said.

High cholesterol shouldn't be ignored, but it's not the only thing that matters. You have to look at the whole picture and consider everything—not just numbers on a readout.

- Protect your liver by:
- Limiting or avoiding refined grains and refined sugars
- Eating fruits and vegetables and take the Heal and Recovery powder every day
- Eating soluble fiber found in legumes, fruits, vegetables, nuts, seeds, psyllium, and whole grains
- Replacing unhealthy fats with healthy fats such as avocados and healthy oils; olive, coconut, avocado, and fish
- Exercising regularly and include resistance training
- Maintaining a healthy weight ratio
- Making sure you stay hydrated

LIE NUMBER 3: FATS ARE FATS. LET'S TAKE A CLOSER LOOK.

For years we have been taught that a low-fat diet is how you lose weight and stay healthy. An entire generation was raised on a low-fat diet, and look where that got us (we are one of the world's sickest countries). Low-fat diets are a half-truth. High-fat diets have been proven, through research, to be far superior to low-fat diets. You need to eat the right type of fats and avoid fats that are responsible for adding belly fat and are a significant contributor to high blood pressure, high cholesterol, cancer, heart disease, digestive issues, diabetes, and many other diseases.

Try to avoid these seven fats:

1. Margarine and butter substitutes
2. Cottonseed oil
3. Corn oil
4. Hydrogenated and partially hydrogenated oils (vegetable oils)
5. Peanut oil
6. Soybean oil
7. Safflower oil

These fats are hidden in many foods that aren't even considered "fattening." To reiterate, the fats that I recommend are in avocados and healthy oils such as olive, coconut, avocado, and fish.

LIFE APPLICATION SECTION

Memory Verse

And the priest shall burn them on the altar as food, an offering made by fire for a sweet aroma; all the fat is the LORD's.

—Leviticus 3:16

Reflections

1. What is the number on one big fat lie most are told about fat?

_____

_____

_____

_____

2. Write down three examples of good fats.

_____

_____

_____

_____

12

IT PAYS TO TREAT, NOT TO CURE!

D DID YOU KNOW THAT THE AVERAGE ANNUAL COST spent on health in America today has nearly tripled in the last 15 years? According to the most recent data available from the Centers for Medicare and Medicaid Services (CMS), the average spending on health-related necessities today for a family of four is $25,826 per year, compared to the annual average of $8,414 in 2001. Add that to the cost of prescription medications – which account for almost 17 percent of all health care spending across the country – and it's easy to see that people are paying more money to fix health problems than to prevent them in the first place.

Health insurance is not preventative; it is reactive! The staggering costs of insurance are in no way helping you remain healthy. Instead, these costly premiums only truly benefit a family member when he or she falls ill. And even then, the average insurance plan seldom covers the entire cost, leaving family after family paying out of pocket for remaining treatments, surgeries, and medicines.

So What's The Alternative?

What if there was another way to control your health and protect your body from sickness and disease? A way that didn't involve endless paperwork and fruitless payments? There is! Rather than be tied down to payment plans that will only bode well for if you fall ill, release yourself from the shackles of health insurance by adopting a healthy lifestyle! When fed and nourished by the proper nutrition and adequately hydrated, the body can be miraculous and self-healing, the way God designed it to be! Prevention is the key to excellent health! An optimal diet and lifestyle will almost totally eliminate the risk of disease. That is not my opinion!

I have realized that many people drift through life—never reaching out for anything. Never choosing a dream and going for it, but simply drifting. And for most people, they also drift with their health. And just like sands in an hourglass, one, by one, by one, their life just slips into the history books. And as the book of their life begins to close, they will wonder to themselves, "What would my life have been if I would have taken my health seriously?"

Sometimes the job of a coach is to "wake people up." Waking people up to the reality that they are health drifting and that there is so much more out there, waiting for them when they get healthy! And the first step towards getting healthy is "giving yourself permission to change!"

The beautiful thing is that WE ALL CAN MAKE THE CHOICE TO CHANGE!

Is there work you need to do which you have been putting off? Is there a trip you've wanted to take, but your physical condition makes it impossible? Is there some shared experience or memory you want to create with a loved one or a friend? Do not wait any longer; do it now. NOW is the time to decide that you are going to get healthy and be the REAL you!

What are the main reasons why people experience health drift? The first reason is we are unprepared as we move from our growing years to our non-growing years. There are metabolic changes and shifts as we go through life. Our growing years may last until we are twenty years old. Our metabolism is at its highest during our growing years, and we are burning those calories at our highest rate. How many times have you heard, "I could eat as much as I wanted when I was younger." During that time, habits and eating styles are being created. Our metabolism changes when we stop growing, but if our habits do not change, we begin adding weight. This weight gain can happen each year at a very steady rate.

Women will point out how metabolism changes after pregnancy, giving birth, and the hormonal changes their bodies go through. These changes are not able to support the same type of habits and eating style. One of the keys is to be willing to make adjustments as the body changes.

Or there are life changes. Life is much different when we are young; playing and active, or a high school athlete who has coaches and parents "making" them do certain things that promote healthier living. After college, it can be finding a job, getting married, and having children; as personal responsibilities increase, the focus and time available to take care of personal health decreases.

Yet, I think the reason why so many people "health drift" is because as the years pass, they are deep down, afraid of permitting themselves to truly change. They are afraid of opening up their lives to what it will take to make lifestyle modifications and truly listen to that small, still voice that has been urging you to GO! But remember that we only have today. Tomorrow is not guaranteed.

If we keep putting off listening until tomorrow… one tomorrow will turn into two, which will turn into three, which will turn into a thousand. And before you know it, you will be at the end of your life, swimming in an ocean of regret. Never forget, at whatever stage of life you are in, good health will only enhance every dream or desire you have, while poor health can and usually will limit those same dreams and desires.

🍎

Don't fall victim to "health drift" – take charge of your life, TODAY!

"Today is all we have.
Today is our gift.
Today is the only time in which we can say 'yes.'
Not yesterday. Not tomorrow. Only today."

There is no doubt that being fit spiritually is the most important kind of health. But being healthy physically is very important too. Many people know the Bible and have a great relationship with God - they pray regularly and have strong faith, but they don't have the physical health or energy to be the person God has created them to be.

All three parts of our being -mental, physical, and spiritual should be healthy and balanced for us to function at optimal levels. Our body is the temple of the Holy Spirit, and we are responsible for how we treat it. So seek balance, try to be healthy, and honor God with all three parts of our life.

You see, when we honor God with our mind, body, and spirit, He will honor us! The Bible says in Deuteronomy 28:2, "His blessings will chase you down and overtake you." That means you will receive blessings that you didn't even earn or deserve!!! That's God rewarding you for walking in faith and honoring Him by taking care of your temple.

I am reminded of the story of Ruth in the Old Testament. She was gathering up the leftover wheat that the workers in the field had missed. She was faithful to her mother-in-law, Naomi, but they were struggling to make ends meet. The owner of the fields (Boaz) told his workers to leave handfuls of wheat behind for Ruth. Ruth came into blessings that she didn't earn or deserve. But because of her faithfulness, God lined up Boaz to be her blessing.

Just look at your life, and you can begin to see times where God has dropped unexpected blessings and provisions that you didn't earn or deserve. Stay in faith and keep being faithful with your temple because you deserve to be the best and highest version of yourself!

LIFE APPLICATION SECTION

Memory Verse

Now a certain woman had a flow of blood for twelve years, [26] and had suffered many things from many physicians. She had spent all that she had and was no better, but rather grew worse.

—Mark 5:25-26

Reflections

1. What do we mean when we say, "Health insurance is not preventative; it is reactive?"

_____

_____

_____

_____

2. Why is prevention the key to excellent health?

_____

_____

_____

_____

But don't be so concerned about perishable things like food. Spend your energy seeking the eternal life that the Son of Man can give you. For God the Father has given me the seal of his approval."

John 6:27

13

SAY NO TO DRUGS!

M OST OF US HAVE NEEDED A PRESCRIPTION OR over-the-counter medication at some point in our lives to treat an infection, disease, psychological condition, or pain.

While some medications can provide lifesaving benefits, sometimes we have to ask if their risks outweigh those benefits.

According to the Mayo Clinic, approximately seven in ten Americans take prescription drugs, with antibiotics, antidepressants, and painkiller opioids among the most common prescriptions given. Meanwhile, 20% of American adults are on five or more prescription medications daily. These medications contain several side effects, including depleting the body of iron, zinc, selenium, and magnesium. This is especially concerning since most Americans already suffer from a nutrient deficiency, leading to chronic disease.

Nutrients are essential to the metabolic activities of every cell in the body. They are consumed in the process and need to be replaced by new nutrients in food or supplements. Depletions occur as some medications block the absorption, storage, metabolism, or synthesis of essential nutrients in the body's gastrointestinal tract, while others deplete by speeding up the metabolic rate. Some medications act as appetite suppressants that can deprive the body of vital nutrients, while other medications increase the desire for unhealthy foods. Many mental health medications can cause insulin resistance resulting in blood sugar swings and increased prevalence of metabolic syndrome.

Antibiotics can eliminate harmful bacteria from the body. They can also deplete the GI tract of good gut bacteria, resulting in digestion problems, including diarrhea, bloating, and gas, as well as yeast infections and colitis. We can counteract these effects with probiotics or fermented foods like unsweetened yogurt and kefir and cultured vegetables like sauerkraut.

Antacids neutralize the stomach's pH and decrease the absorption of iron and folic acid, and zinc. Weight loss drugs and cholesterol-lowering agents bind to healthy fats and prevent them from being absorbed. For example, widely prescribed "statin" drugs block HMG-CoA activity, an enzyme required to manufacture cholesterol in the body. This action also depletes the body of coenzyme Q10 (CoQ10), resulting in a serious and negative impact on muscle and cardiovascular health.

You should always talk to your doctor or pharmacist and review all of your medications to see if one or more might be depleting nutrients from your bodies. If both of these health professionals are not sure, you may need laboratory tests to look for deficiencies. Following the LT360 lifestyle and the recommended quality supplementation can overcome and prevent serious health issues caused by these nutrient deficiencies.

People being prescribed these drugs have very little to do with our doctors or health care providers. It's about how our health care, or should I say sick care system is set up.

I've spoken many times on the history of how our current healthcare system is broken. The bottom line is that we are the best at treating infections and trauma, but we are among the worst in preventing chronic illness and diseases.

For example, if you get your arm cut off in an accident or you get the flu, we are in the greatest health care system in the world. But what it doesn't do well is deal with chronic health issues, prevention, and getting to the "why?" or the underlying cause of the malady. And so we have become experts in masking symptoms. In doing so, we might reduce or eliminate that symptom temporarily, but we are also likely causing more significant harm by not understanding the cause of the symptoms in the first place.

I've heard it described as a game of "Whack-a-Mole" where you treat one symptom, and then your body pops up with another symptom, and you take another medication until another symptom appears, and then the game starts all over again. The problem with this approach is that it hasn't gotten your body back to a state where it has healed and repaired itself and can operate without some drug indefinitely.

As the old saying goes, "An ounce of prevention is worth a pound of cure."

The next problem is sick care vs. health care. You've probably noticed the system only gets paid when you get sick. If you stay healthy, they make a lot less money. The more treatments or drugs you take, the more you pay. Our healthcare system is incentivized by treating symptoms instead of the core root causes and enabling the body to heal and repair itself through a natural, non-invasive approach; if they did, the money would disappear very quickly.

We want to believe in our doctors; we are brought up and led to believe they are the "experts." Yes, they are highly respected in our culture, and there are good reasons why; the education and training alone they receive is extensive. A closer look, though, reveals they are not trained or experts in the areas of wellness and nutrition. I can't tell you how many times I have heard from a doctor how they took only one nutrition class during the entire educational process. Interestingly, when we know many foods, based on their nutritional value, possess strong healing properties. It is not a criticism, but they do not generally have the expertise in those areas; their expertise lies elsewhere.

When we have a body with tremendous healing and regenerative properties but are prescribed certain medications,

especially long term, it creates a huge problem. That is one of those instances where what we are doing is actually working against the body instead of working with the body. I can't tell you how many clients have shared one of the main goals of becoming aLT360 client: the strong desire to get off or at least reduce their medications. They realize what the medications are doing to their body and overall health; that the side effects become more dangerous than the disorder for which it was prescribed.

Of course, we don't make medical claims or guarantee that anyone will get off their medications. Regardless of how confident we are, by law, we cannot make those types of claims. Plus, we leave any decisions related to those medications between you and your doctor. Yet, why are there so many testimonies of those getting off or reducing their medications? One must only go back to the premise. I repeat, the body has excellent healing and regenerative powers, and when you work with it, your body will work with you. That is "the why," and when your WHY for getting healthy becomes stronger than those things you are currently allowing yourself to be distracted with, excellent outcomes are in store.

LIFE APPLICATION SECTION

Memory Verse

They gave Him sour wine mingled with gall to drink. But when He had tasted it, He would not drink.

—Matthew 27:34

Reflections

1. Nutrients are essential to the metabolic activities of what organ in the body?

_____

_____

_____

_____

2. Why are so many doctors simply drug pushers?

_____

_____

_____

_____

14

SUPPLEMENTS VS. DRUGS

SINCE GETTING STARTED WITH MY JOURNEY, I HAVE known some supplements could help and accelerate the process of getting healthy at the cellular level. What started merely as recommendations have evolved into a full-fledged approach of having a natural, holistic supplement to recommend in place of any prescribed medication. This initially happened because there were so many options for even a single vitamin, I wanted to become a trusted source with fair pricing. With so many people needing and desiring to come off or reduce their medications, I wanted to meet those needs and desires. It has grown from making supplement recommendations to a full line of supplements with our HEAL products, designed to prevent and reverse chronic illnesses and disease.

Some people have asked why do you need supplements if you are eating a healthy diet? So here is a good way to understand the importance of supplements from my friends at myhdiet.com.

Our fruits and vegetables are not as nutritious as they once were.

Modern farming practices, such as the heavy use of fertilizers, pesticides, and other substances, have resulted in soil that is almost sterile and devoid of trace minerals. As a result, our food is not as nutritious as it was decades ago. In a recent review on modern foods, scientists found that the larger the crop yield, the lower the mineral concentration.

Furthermore, a historical analysis of the nutritional composition of fruits and vegetables has confirmed a decline in several nutrients over the last 50-70 years. Specifically, hybrid versions of broccoli, wheat, and corn have also shown lower mineral content.

As you age, your body changes how it processes food and needs or nutritional support.

In our older years, we need almost as many nutrients as we did in our youth, but we don't burn as many calories. To compensate for this, we need to maximize the nutrients we consume in each calorie. We also need to make sure our bodies are fully fed at the cellular level. This is also where superfoods and "concentrated" foods like fresh vegetable juice help, as you get an abundance of vegetables in a form the body can readily absorb.

Supplements are to "add to" eating healthy;
they are not a substitute for it!

Supplements help us ease or counteract specific health conditions we encounter throughout our lifetimes.

We each have unique weaknesses, conditions, or stages in life that put additional strain on us. Sometimes, there are supplements to help us get through these times until we heal and recover. Although the quantity and type of nutrients consumed varies from person to person, no one can rely on a healthy diet alone to effectively stave off diseases, detoxify and live as energetically and vibrantly as possible.

Certain nutrients aren't available in optimal amounts through diet alone—regardless of the type of diet.

For example, MSM or Methylsulfonylmethane and Vitamin C, which are in the HEAL & Recovery Powder, are the miracle supplements our bodies can't get enough of. Many of our clients take the HEAL & Recovery Powder every day, and why I recommend it to all my patients.

I hope this helps you understand the importance of supplementation. Now let me talk about a few of our HEAL products and why I am recommending them:

HEAL AND RECOVERY

As we age, our bodies go through some normal wear and tear in the process. And because of this, additional nutritional support is beneficial and necessary. The best nutrition for your body's ability to heal and repair itself are those responsible for energy production, cell growth, repair, and hydration; these are found in the HEAL and Recovery Powder (H/R).

H/R Powder is designed to strengthen the body's systems on a cellular level by regulating growth, immune system functions, and metabolism that keep the body's cells functioning at an optimal level. When it comes to quality and efficacious results, H/R is a proven winner.

Our bodies are designed to absorb and utilize the natural ingredients in bio-active ingredients to strengthen the body's systems on a cellular level by regulating growth, immune system functions, and metabolism that keep the body's cells functioning at an optimal level. A good source I highly recommend is Healing and Recovery Powder (www.foodwars.org/Products).

Some of the health benefits include:

- o   Anti-inflammatory effects
- o   Strengthening the immune system
- o   Supporting healthy digestion and nutrient absorption

Here are a few of the many nutritional ingredients from HEAL and Recovery: that should be a staple in your supplement pantry:

MSM or Methylsulfonylmethane

MSM is an organic sulfur compound that plays a critical role in energy production within every cell of the body. MSM can assist in the manufacture of ATP, the energy molecule that fuels cells. This means you'll have more available energy for your workouts and daily activities. What makes MSM one of the best and most unique supplements is its ability to impact cell health in more ways than one. MSM helps regulate inflammation on a cell- by-cell basis, which is excellent for muscles engaging in strenuous activity. It also is an excellent antioxidant protecting cells from free radical damage while helping clear out toxins in the body.

Read your supplement labels, avoid those with a lot of filler ingredients.

Vitamin C

Vitamin C offers multiple health benefits, making it one of the best vitamins for workouts. Vitamin C has antioxidant properties that prevent free radical materials from damaging the body's cells. Free radicals are by-products that form when cells convert food into energy. Since obviously working out burns energy, healthy vitamin C levels can prevent these harmful materials from building up in the cells. Vitamin C also helps repair and rebuild cells and tissues, such as muscles, ligaments, and tendons. Repair and rebuilding processes are necessary for improved strength and performance. In effect, healthy levels of vitamin C allow the body to reap the full benefits of exercise.

Tart Cherry

Tart Cherry contains smaller amounts of B vitamins, calcium, iron, magnesium, omega-3, and omega-6 fats, in addition to antioxidants and other beneficial plant compounds. Tart cherry has also been shown to reduce muscle breakdown, muscle soreness and speed up recovery times.

Turmeric

Turmeric can be a powerful tool in the fight against obesity and its related symptoms, as shown in research. Turmeric reduces leptin resistance, lowers insulin resistance, reverses hyperglycemia, reduces inflammation, and activates fat-burning gene signals. And these are only a few of the great things that this spice can do.

Vitamin D3

Vitamin D3can help lower your blood pressure. Suppose you're trying to reduce your risk of diabetes or lower your chances of heart attacks, rheumatoid arthritis, or multiple sclerosis. In that case, vitamin D should be part of your daily supplements. According to Michael F. Holick, Ph.D., MD, head of the Vitamin D, Skin, and Bone Research Laboratory at Boston University School of Medicine, Vitamin D also helps regulate your immune system and can be a potent inhibitor of cancer cell growth.

HEAL and Recovery

H/R is one of the very few supplements that can be as effective as a drug. As you can see, daily use of the above supplements has powerful effects on many aspects of health at the cellular level. And best of all, they may also be helpful as a shield of protection against chronic illness and disease, as well as an anti- aging supplement while building your immune system.

HEAL Multi-Collagen and Gut Restore

The game of health starts in your gut! Did you know that more than 70% of your immune system is housed in your gut? So when it comes to staying healthy, gut health isn't only about avoiding nasty digestive problems. It's a critical part of your overall wellness of being active, enjoying the time with your family and friends, and having enough strength and energy to do what you want to do without being held back at every point by the "bubble guts" and digestive discomfort.

That's why our multi-collagen protein has 1 billion CPU of soil-based probiotics that promote a healthy gut microflora, reduces occasional bloating, and supports healthy skin, hair, and nails. This product contains the three ingredients of the Gut Health "TRIPLE DOUBLE:" Prebiotics, Probiotics, and Postbiotics.

Here's why each is important.

1. Prebiotics are the food for the beneficial bacteria in your gut.
   For these good bacteria to be as helpful as possible, they need food. And prebiotics gives them what they need to thrive. Common prebiotics includes fiber and other types of carbs that humans don't easily digest. These bacteria eat this fiber, which helps to support the balance in your gut.

2. Probiotics are beneficial bacteria in your gut.

These are the bacteria themselves and support healthy digestion and digestive function. They make the journey to your gut, and then they help support it in multiple ways. One way they help support your gut is by promoting the balance of beneficial bacteria.

3. Postbiotics are the result of probiotics eating prebiotics.

This process and production of postbiotics have many health- boosting functions. These postbiotics are the "result" of effective probiotics—and they're responsible for many of the beneficial effects we see from taking probiotics.

HEAL Cannabidiol (CBD) Oil

Many people think that hemp and marijuana are two different species of plant. But the truth is they're not distinct species. They're just two different names for cannabis, found in the Cannabaceae family. The main difference between the two is tetrahydrocannabinol (THC) content. CBD is 100% legal.

1. Physical Benefits of CBD

CBD stimulates an anti-inflammatory response that helps reduce all forms of chronic aches and pains. Regular use also helps support joint health, mobility, and flexibility.

2. Psychological Benefits

It helps positively regulate mood patterns which help reduce anxiety, stress, and feeling overwhelmed. It also promotes better sleep cycles and can offer a safe, all-natural remedy for depression and bipolar disorders.

3. Neurological Benefits

CBD can help reduce age-related cognitive decline and memory loss. It also helps support focus, alertness, and memory recall while reducing the frequency of migraines and headaches.

The problem with CBD oil has been that it has been unregulated, so it is difficult to determine the quality of the product and even if it is an authentic CBD product in the first place. However, LT360's CBD Oil is organically grown, certified, and third-party tested for potency, purity, and efficacy. That is a must for anyone to be confident in the CBD product purchased.

HEAL 5 Star Omega Fish Oil

LT360's 5 Star Omega fish oil has unsurpassed benefits in terms of supporting a healthy heart, the brain, the immune system, eyes, joints, and moods. 5 Star Omega Fish Oil will provide you with marine lipid concentrate that has been processed by molecular distillation while also providing omega-3 fatty acids, including eicosapentaenoic acid (EPA, 18%) and docosahexaenoic acid (DHA, 12%), in their triglyceride form, which is lacking in the American diet. When researching the best omega three oils, look for a concentration of DHA, the most important of all Omega-3 oils and one that is safe from heavy metals or anything artificial. You also want one that does not have a fishy taste. One that fits that bill is 5-Star Omega Fish Oil.

Fish Oil is known to treat health issues including heart disease, ADHD, anxiety, depression, high cholesterol, inflammatory bowel disease, Alzheimer's disease, eczema, diabetes, cancer, weakened immunity, autoimmune disease, and macular degeneration. It's been proven to aid the body in weight loss, fertility, healthy pregnancy, healthy skin, and increased energy.

These are simply a few of the supplement options we recommend. The more you understand what each does and the benefit to your overall health, the better you can understand their importance in our current culture based on the current American diet.

LIFE APPLICATION SECTION

Memory Verse

"Please test your servants for ten days, and let them give us vegetables to eat and water to drink. [13] Then let our appearance be examined before you, and the appearance of the young men who eat the portion of the king's delicacies; and as you see fit, so deal with your servants."

—Daniel 1:12-13

Reflections

1. What is the difference between supplements and drugs?

_____

_____

_____

_____

2. What ailments is fish oil known to treat?

_____

_____

_____

_____

Then the LORD said to Moses,
"Take fragrant spices--gum resin,
onycha, and galbanum--and pure
frankincense, all in equal amounts,
and make a fragrant blend of incense,
the work of a perfumer. It is to be
salted and pure and sacred.

Genesis 30:35-36

15

WHY FAD DIETS ARE DANGEROUS, AND DON'T WORK!

I HAVE TRIED EVERY DIET KNOWN TO MAN. THESE include weight watchers, Jenny Craig, Nutrisystem, Adkins, pills, powders, potions, and lotions, and I could go on, but you get the picture. The point is fad diets have been around for many decades. But beyond a temporary fix, a fad diet typically promotes some "magic" pill, powder, potion, or lotion that excludes certain essential nutrients and encourages following other unnecessary rules to focus on changing your body chemistry to lose weight fast. Since fad diets are designed as a temporary "fix" for quick and often unhealthy weight loss, you cannot create what is needed: a permanent lifestyle change based on consistency (not perfection).

And as many of us have found out, not only do these diets fail to work long term, they can also be dangerous. This is because these radical fad diets often cut out essential nutritional foods that you need for overall health and wellness at the cellular level.

Remember, the body is designed for survival. When you begin to do things too restrictive or too intense, the alarm bells begin to ring, and the body switches to survival mode. The fat- releasing process actually begins to slow down instead of speeding up. That is why in the long run, diets that are too restrictive or too intense in fact train the body to store fat. Thus, many people proclaim how easy it was to gain it all back. A deprived body will grab and hold faster than you can imagine when given a chance.

Here are a few examples of fad diets:

1. Low-fat diet
2. Liquid protein diet
3. All-cabbage diet
4. Grapefruit diet
5. Low carb or no carb diet
6. HCG diet and many others

All diets promise weight loss but fail to mention that the pounds shed are most often just water weight, which is another reason why you'll end up gaining it back as soon as you stop following their plan. Another thing that is not mentioned is that you won't get the calories, vitamins, and minerals you need to thrive and get healthy at the cellular level.

While some of these diets may seem harmless, it all comes back to one principle: these dietary restrictions won't have all of the essential nutrients your body needs to function at the highest level. Anna King, a registered dietitian at Riley Hospital for Children at Indiana University Health, says, "Each food group provides its own unique set of vitamins, minerals, and energy for the body." That is why we need a variety of macro and micro nutrition that a balanced diet will provide. This is excellent advice and sound teaching.

It's time to stop dieting! When you change your mind about your health, your body will follow.

You see, your body cannot function at the optimal level without a variety of essential vitamins, minerals, and nutrients. With the proper nutrition, you can boost your energy, strengthen your immune system, get adequately hydrated, reduce your risk for developing chronic illness and disease, improve your mental health, and promote longevity, all while being the person you were created to be.

That's why having a framework to work with the way your body is designed is always better than a short-term fad diet. Following the LT360 plan will allow you to take back control of your life and treat your body the way God intended you to care for it – with love and proper nourishment.

Stop believing that those fad diets are the best option for you. It's time to get healthy at the cellular level and live your best life now!!!

Most people know that it is important to be proactive in preventing serious diseases and illnesses such as cancer and heart disease: but they get overwhelmed by the mass quantity of information available regarding health and wellness. Instead of getting caught up in the complicated details, it is much easier to take it back to the basics. Getting back to the basics that will work is how LT360 has been designed.

One of the most basic principles is learning to work with your BMR (Basic Metabolic Rate). BMR is the number of calories your body will use in a 24-hour calorie expenditure day. There are impedance technology scales that can let you know what your BMR is, and there are formulas based on gender, height, and weight that are available online where it can be calculated. The answer is usually based on a typical day, and then adjustments can be made on how many calories your body needs and uses based on a day with activity (+10%) or a "couch potato" day (-10%)

It would help if you always remembered, whether you consciously count calories or not, your body is always counting. It does not mean you always have to count calories and make a note of each one. But you will need and must have the proper framework in place (e.g.,

LT360) and become very intuitive with how your body responds to certain foods and meals. The result will provide the awareness you will need.

Remember, if you consistently overeat your BMR, you give your body only one choice, STORE IT AS FAT. If your body can't use those calories, it must store them. How quickly can a person gain weight? Consistently eating only 100 calories above and beyond your BMR per day (which is extremely easy to do and not even noticeable) equals a gain of close to 1 lb. per month or 10- 12 lbs. per year. Do you see how easy it is to have that "10 lb."

weight creep each year? Once you get the LT360 5 to Thrive framework in place, the key is to accept and work with your BMR. BMR is very different for each individual, and you have no other choice but to work (or not work) with yours if you want to get back in balance and be healthy.

A person's eating style is a critical component in creating a person's healthy lifestyle. Learning and having the discipline to not turn to food and eating during times when it becomes more harmful than good is essential. Examples of "harmful" eating are during high times of emotion, stress, depression, or anxiety. Food has the intended purpose of providing energy; however, eating while highly emotional or highly stressed will generally equate to overeating.

You may not count calories, but your body is always counting!

Of course, it would be nice during life's "happenings," during those times of high emotion and/or stress, the body would do each of us a favor and burn more calories, but it is not the way it works. Since it does not work that way, it all boils down to whether someone is willing to work with his or her BMR (do you see the theme here?). So, if you are an emotional or stress eater, continue to find alternatives and positive ways to deal with those times instead of turning to food.

I also want to strongly caution you not to continue to use emotional eating as an excuse. Realize the time to go to battle with this eating style to create a new and better approach to eating is now. How do you know if you are simply using stress and life happening as an excuse is now to eat? One way to determine if you are using stress as an excuse to eat is to consider if you think about whether you are eating out of an emotional state before or after the fact? Giving in to the "I have always been this way" mindset can quickly become an excuse.

Allowing yourself to have this eating style is a very deceptive way not to take personal responsibility and accountability. Using it as an excuse can allow you to find a way to remove it from you and place it outside of yourself into the category of "life circumstances."

Yes, it will be a battle, possibly an all-out war, one you are capable of winning, but you must begin by treating it as such. Do you know the type of person I have never met? One who is happy with him or herself by being an emotional eater.

If you are an emotional eater, you know it's rarely about food but the feelings connected to the food. And that connection can be very unhealthy. So the question is, what feeling is the enemy using to keep you hooked on emotional eating?

Do you remember the old school song, "Hooked on a Feeling?" The 1968 pop song was written by Mark James and originally performed by B.J. Thomas. If you do, then you remember the lyrics that say, "I'm hooked on a feeling!" Similarly, the enemy has used food to "HOOK" us on our feelings connected to food.

Here is where the lie starts and the deception begins:

    ♧Joy ÆPeace ♧Love ♧Comfort ♧Belonging And all of
    these emotions became the "Hook!"

You need to recognize that the enemy is a great deceiver, and he knows the hooks he needs to reinforce our behavior which is the lure to reeling us in.

Scripture describes the enemy as "cunning." The definition of cunning is "having or showing skill in achieving one's ends by deceit or evasion." But God makes us a promise concerning temptation in 1 Corinthians 10:13, *"No temptation has overtaken you except such as is common to man; but God is faithful, who will not allow you to be tempted beyond what you are able, but with the temptation will also make the way of escape, that you may be able to bear it."* YES! YES! YES! So, the next time the enemy uses a "food lure" to trap you in your feelings, reflect on God's promise and His love for you. Begin today to choose life, not the lure!

That is why you must make a lifestyle choice, not a diet choice. It is why LT360 is not a diet but a program. You must find a framework to help you create a lifestyle, to be an overcomer. I do not know of any healthy person who does not have a healthy lifestyle based on a consistent, healthy routine.

Keep in mind that small changes in your daily habits can directly impact your overall health and wellness. Even though these small decisions might seem mundane, it is worth the effort because those choices will add up in the long run.

LIFE APPLICATION SECTION

Memory Verse

There is a way that seems right to a man, but its end is the way of death.

—Proverbs 14:12

Reflections

1. Why don't fad diets work?

_____

_____

_____

_____

2. Why is it important to get healthy at a cellular level?

_____

_____

_____

_____

16

"5 TO THRIVE: THE UNIVERSAL HEALTH SOLUTION"

AS A COACH, I HAVE ALWAYS TAUGHT FUNDAMENTALS. so let's start with the basics of cellular health. We call it the "5 TO THRIVE!" Use these five simple strategies that you can always count on and implement to boost your health in a sustainable way.

1. Hydration
2. Fasted Exercise
3. Meal Timing and Multiple Smaller Meals
4. Reading Food Labels
5. Sleep – Make it a Priority

Now, let's look at each of these strategies more closely.

1. HYDRATION

The simplest and cost-effective way to get healthy is to drink more water. I have encouraged our patients to build up to drinking 1/2 their body weight in ounces a day. As long as you have healthy kidneys, then it is a good target. I always say that a hydrated cell is a healthy cell. Just think about it this way, what is the difference between a grape and a raisin? That's right, hydration.

2. FASTED EXERCISE

I recommend 30-45 minutes a day of moderate exercise between 4-5 days a week. I also recommend first thing in the morning on an empty stomach. Many people have asked me why I exercise on an empty stomach and why we teach it as part of the 5 to Thrive. So here is my take and some of the science and research to support these strategies.

Working out on an empty stomach or what is known as training in a fasting state improves several physiological markers that are especially important to people with type 2 diabetes, high blood pressure, and cholesterol issues. First of all, it improves insulin sensitivity. Simply put, type 2 diabetes is "extreme insulin resistance," and moderate fasted workouts can drastically improve insulin resistance. It also improves fat burning, another deficiency common in people with type 2 diabetes. People suffering from HBP (high blood pressure) and cholesterol issues seem to do better in the fasted state.

When you exercise on an empty stomach, you can rapidly improve body composition and your muscles' ability to burn fat. Research shows that both men and women saw better VO2max increases when they exercised in a fasted state, boosting muscle oxidative capacity. VO_2 max refers to how much oxygen your body can absorb and use during exercise. This is excellent news when you are trying to lose fat and gain lean muscle! Studies also show considerable gains in hydration over time as well.

Now, always keep in mind that we are talking about moderate forms of exercise and resistance training. If you are training with high levels of intense training or preparing to run a marathon, eating before training is advised.

Resistance Training

The best advice I received from my coach was to maintain resistance training throughout my life. It is something I have always remembered. So, I have recommended resistance bands for 10-minutes a day for 4-5 days a week.

We know that developing lean muscle is the secret to long- term metabolic boosting. The great news is that you don't have to tie a rope around your waist and drag a 50 lb kettlebell across the parking lot, and flip tires overall day to be fit and develop some lean muscle. You can do this at any level and age.

After almost two decades of coaching high-performance athletes on how to get bigger, faster, and stronger, I realized one thing, I was wrong! I used to teach them that you have to go heavy and hard with more reps if you want to get stronger. Although there is some truth to that, I've learned that you can increase strength without necessarily killing yourself and hating the process with heavy weights. The best part? The strategies that I teach require minimal equipment and no gym membership, as it is all about technique, not crazy weight loads. Slow it down and use the negative accentuated movements.

That is, one second positive (pull or push movement), five- seven second negative (releasing the pull or push movement. A simple change in tempo will add more tension to every rep and set, increasing the amount of muscle fibers being called upon. Once you get to the maintenance phase, you can adjust your strategy slightly and perhaps speed up your reps with good technique.

A key is to improve your form. I am often asked, "Coach, how can I go to the next level in my lean muscle development?" My answer is always the same, Perfect your technique first, then move to other exercises. When you improve and progress your technique over time, it's incredible how your body will respond.

3. MEAL TIMING AND MULTIPLE SMALLER MEALS

"Timing is EVERYTHING." When you eat multiple, smaller meals with consistency, even if you don't feel hungry, you are getting ahead of the low blood sugar drops and controlling your blood sugar during the active part of your day. Now, with our schedules so disrupted, many of us need to "re-set our eating clocks." This helps re-engage our metabolism.

We all know the feeling when we skip meals in the morning or skip lunch. We get famished by 3 pm or 4 pm, and we start looking around for something to snack on. Most of the time, it is sweet or salty carbs. And some people skip meals altogether and say, "I'll just wait for dinner." Am I talking to anyone yet? Now you have put your body into severe low blood sugar, and you start snacking the minute you get home, or maybe going way over your caloric ranges at dinner. You are not alone! This happens to everyone at some point in their life. But this habit can keep you from getting healthy and reaching your goals.

As disruptive as it is to your metabolism during the day (it stalls out your energy levels), it also signals or communicates to the body that you are starving. Our bodies read this low blood sugar as: "There may not be enough food out there, better HOLD ON to the stored fat."

On the other hand, if blood sugar is successfully managed during the day, the body reads it as: "Times are good - we don't need all of these energy reserves (fat), I will get fed again tomorrow!" This is exactly why weight loss may have been unsuccessful before; in an attempt to EAT LESS, you have communicated to your body NOT to lose weight.

Eating smaller meals four-five times a day can be AS important as the FOOD itself. Frequency, along with protein and the reduction of refined grains and sugars, helps manage blood sugar in your active phase, giving your body PERMISSION to release stored fat as food or fuel. Try and eat every three-four hours.

4. READING FOOD LABELS

Having a basic understanding of product labels and using them to make good meal choices I critical. Consider this example of a label for frozen lasagna:[8]

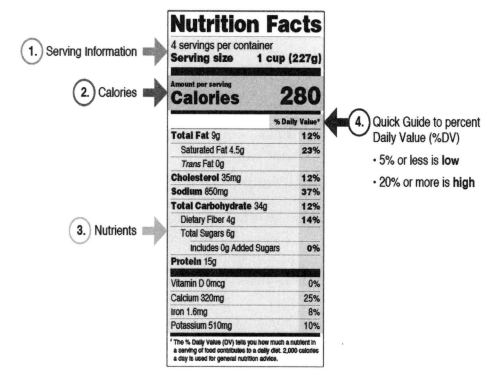

A. Don't Let the Claims on the Front Packaging Fool You

One of the best tips may be to completely ignore claims on the front of the packaging. For example, what are these claims saying (or not saying)?

1. **Organic.** This label says nothing about whether a product has no white flour or low in added sugars.

2. **Sugar-Free / No Added Sugar.** Sugar substitutes you need to avoid may have been added.

3. **Made with Whole Grains.** The product may contain very little whole grains. Check the ingredients list — if whole grains aren't in the first three ingredients, the amount is negligible. Also, remember that "wheat flour" or "enriched wheat flour" = the white flour we're avoiding, and when they list this in the ingredients, they are simply informing us that the flour is made from the grain in the field named wheat, and not made from corn or rice or something else.

B. Ingredients List

Product ingredients are listed by weight — from highest to lowest amount. The ingredients list does NOT inform us of the individual amount of each listed item in the product. Instead, the nutrition chart gives us an indication of that. Review the ingredients list for items you choose to avoid, such as wheat flour (the white flour we're avoiding), artificial sweeteners, etc.

C. Nutrition Chart

Review the nutrition chart for the amount of added sugars and the protein grams per serving size you will consume, keeping in mind our meal targets of 9g or fewer added sugars and 20-25+g protein.

1. **Serving information:** First, look at the number of servings in the package (servings per container) and the serving size. The serving size reflects the amount people typically eat or drink. ***IT IS NOT A RECOMMENDATION OF HOW MUCH YOU SHOULD EAT OR DRINK. FOR EXAMPLE, YOU MIGHT CONSUME ½ SERVING, 1 SERVING, OR MORE.*** In the sample label, one serving equals 1 cup. If you ate two cups, you would be consuming two servings. That is two times the calories and nutrients shown in the sample label, so you would need to double the nutrient and calorie amounts and the %DVs to see what you are getting in two servings.

2. **Calories:** Calories provide a measure of how much energy you get from a serving of this food. In the label example above, there are 280 calories in one serving. What if you ate the entire package? Then you would consume four servings or 1,120 calories. ***REMEMBER: THE NUMBER OF SERVINGS YOU CONSUME DETERMINES THE NUMBER OF CALORIES YOU ACTUALLY EAT.***

3. **Nutrients:** Section 3 in the sample label shows some essential nutrients determined to impact health. Use the added sugars line of this section to support our target of keeping our MEAL added sugars grams at 9g added sugars or fewer.

    ADDED sugars on the Nutrition Facts label include sugars added during the processing of foods, including sucrose, dextrose, sugars from syrups and honey, and sugars from concentrated fruit vegetable juices. Note: Having the word "includes" before Added Sugars on the label indicates that Added Sugars are included in the number of grams of sugar.

4. <u>Total Sugars</u>: For example, a product with added sweeteners might list: "Total Sugars 15g", with "Includes 7g Added Sugars" on the line below. That means that the product has 7 grams of Added Sugars and 8 grams of naturally occurring sugars for 15 grams of sugar. As with calories, the number of servings you consume determines the number of added sugars actually eaten. Since natural sugars do not count against you, you only need to count the added sugars.

Reading is fundamental, especially when it comes to nutrition!

D. Percent Daily Value (%DV)

The % Daily Value (%DV) is the percentage of the Daily Value for each nutrient in a serving of the food, or how much of the nutrient in a serving contributes to a total daily diet. For example, a food with 5%DV of a nutrient is considered a low contributor of that nutrient, while 20%DV is considered a high contributor to the daily value of that nutrient.

1. <u>Total Sugars</u>: No Daily Reference Value has been established for Total Sugars because no U.S. recommendations have been made for the total amount to eat in a day. Keep in mind that the Total Sugars listed on the Nutrition Facts label include naturally occurring sugars (like those in fruit and milk) as well as Added Sugars.

2. **Protein:** A %DV is required to be listed if a claim is made for protein, such as "high in protein." The %DV for protein must also be listed on the label if it is intended for infants and children under four years of age. However, if the product is intended for the general population four years of age and older and a claim is not made about protein on the label, the %DV for protein is not required.

E. Protein is non-negotiable.

Protein causes a rise in the thermic effect of food. It increases your metabolism and makes you feel fuller for more extended periods of time, preventing you from overeating. Both animal and plant-based proteins are effective. If you are having trouble getting enough protein in your meals alone, you may want to consider adding a scoop of protein powder to your favorite drink. A good whey or plant-based protein can help you achieve your daily protein goals. I pour my protein drink in my coffee each morning.

Proteins are the building blocks of life; every living cell uses them for structural and functional purposes. There are nine essential amino acids that we must get from the diet and 12 that are non-essential, which the body can produce out of other organic molecules. In this regard, animal proteins are better than plant proteins, which makes perfect sense given that the muscle tissues of animals are very similar to our tissues.

The so-called "health experts" recommend an intake of 56 grams per day for men and 46 grams per day for women, varying between individuals based on age, body weight, activity levels, and other factors. While this minimum intake may be enough to prevent deficiency, it is not sufficient to optimize health and body composition at a cellular level.

Therefore, I recommend shooting for one-half of your body weight in grams of protein per day.

Here are a few quick guidelines from our friends at Institute for Integrative Nutrition:

For vegans: Look for formulas that contain a combination of pea, oat, chia, flax, rice, or hemp proteins. Hemp and chia-based proteins are especially beneficial because they contain all nine essential amino acids, which are the building blocks of protein and necessary for healthy muscle growth.

For Paleo eaters: Whey protein isolate, casein, and egg white protein are all considered Paleo-friendly protein powders.

For gluten-free: If you have a gluten intolerance, be sure to read the label on your protein carefully—some brands contain gluten as a filler. Rice protein or hemp protein powders are typically a safe bet.

5. SLEEP - MAKE IT A PRIORITY

The one-third of our lives that we spend sleeping is far from unproductive. Time spent getting proper sleep plays a direct role in how full, energetic, and successful the other two-thirds of our lives are when we're awake. For example, consider the body's organs and the critical role they play within the body. High-quality sleep supports the kidneys and liver to optimize waste removal and cleansing functions. When asleep, the body will rebuild, cleanse, repair, and re-set the functions that maintain cellular health, protecting a person from illness and disease. Ninety-seven percent of adults need anywhere from seven to nine hours of sleep each night. One study's findings promoted 7 1/2 hours as ideal. A gene mutation identified as gene

DEC2 allows people with the gene to need only 6 hours each night, but this is found in only 3% of the population (abcnews.go.com/Technology). If you are not one of the 3%, then getting less than the required amount of sleep is not training the body to function with less sleep; you are simply becoming sleep-deprived and creating all the issues associated with sleep deprivation.

We must schedule sleep like any other daily activity, so we put it on the "to-do list" and cross it off every night. However, sleep is not the thing to do only after everything else is done. We need to stop doing other things to get the sleep we need.

Make sure to give yourself a chance to get the proper amount of sleep. Remember, everything works together in the 5 to Thrive, and each piece supports the other. As consistency is developed in each of the first four, along with getting the right amount of sleep needed, many find themselves sleeping better and more refreshed when waking up within the first 40 to 60 days.

LIFE APPLICATION SECTION

Memory Verse

So, God split the hollow place that is in Lehi, and water came out, and he drank; and his spirit returned, and he revived. Therefore, he called its name En Hakkore, which is in Lehi to this day.

—Judges 15:19

Reflections

1. Why is hydration critical to getting and living healthy?

2. What is the ideal number of hours of sleep that most adults need each day?

ABOUT THE AUTHORS

Dr. Francis Myles

In 1989, near death, Dr. Myles had a divine encounter with Jesus Christ Himself. After this powerful healing encounter, Dr. Myles was anointed with a strong gift of healing and prophecy. As a result, he has seen thousands of people healed through his crusades and meetings.

Known as a great "revelator." Dr. Myles has been gifted with biblical insight and revelation into many hidden mysteries of the Word. However, he is most well-known for his revelation of the Order of Melchizedek. This revelation has resulted in the creation of "The Order of Melchizedek Supernatural School of Ministry," where he has graduated thousands of students worldwide who have learned the life-changing principles of living as "kings and priests" under this powerful Order.

Dr. Myles is a world-renowned author of many life- changing books such as *The Order of Melchizedek, Issuing Divine Restraining Orders from the Courts of Heaven,* and *The Joseph of Arimethea Calling,* to name just a few. He has made several appearances on TBN, GodTV, and Daystar Christian TV networks. He has been a featured guest on Sid Roth's "Its Supernatural TV show, and This Is Your Day with Benny Hinn."

Dr. Francis Myles is also the founder of Marketplace BibleTM International, the creator of the world's first digital Marketplace Bible, designed to help millions of Christians worldwide to "apply timeless biblical principles to today's marketplace." He is happily married to the love of his life, Carmela Real Myles. Together they reside in McDonough, Georgia, a suburb of Atlanta.

Coach Scott Oatsvall

Coach Scott Oatsvall is the Founder and President of LT360 and LT360 Health Center, a cellular health and integrated health company. LT360 has clients in 29 states and nine foreign countries.

Scott has over 22 years of coaching at the high school and college levels and has been named Coach of the year twice.

He is the host of the "Coaches Health Show" on Super talk 99.7 WTN. He is the author of the book "AND 1," a book that encourages people to experience the miracle of adoption while saying YES to God!

He is also an expert in the field of health, human performance, and personal development. In addition, Scott is a sought-after speaker for his ability to motivate and inspire people to be all they were created to be. Scott speaks to thousands of people each year.

But the most important responsibility in his life belongs to his family. He has been married to his wife, Gwen, for over 30 years. They have two biological sons and four adopted children. They live in Brentwood, Tennessee.

Coach Scott Oatsvall on Facebook
coach@LT360.com
@LT360coach on Twitter and Instagram
www.LT360.com

ENDNOTES

1   htttps://www.healthline.com/health/food-nutrition/
    how-long-can-you-live- without-food#individual-time-period
2   https://www.jewishvirtuallibrary.org/
    rabbinic-teachings-on-vegetarianism
3   http://www.epctoronto.org/Press/Publications_JRHughes/Why_Meat_
    Web. htm
4   https://www.godsaidmansaid.com/topic3.asp?Cat2=244&ItemID=755
5   https://www.forbes.com/sites/niallmccarthy/2017/10/16/u-s-obesity-
    rates- have-hit-an-all-time-high-infographic/#118257044bad
6   https://www.cnbc.com/2017/10/31/fatty-liver-disease-affects-80-
    million- americans.html
7   https://www.cbsnews.com/news/1-in-10-kids-may-have-fatty-livers/
8   https://www.healthline.com/nutrition/how-to-read-food-labels
    https://www.fda.gov/food/new-nutrition-facts-label/
    how-understand-and- use-nutrition-facts-label